simply
sustainable
beauty

**A collection of 50 simple zero waste beauty
recipes to give you naturally beautiful skin & hair**

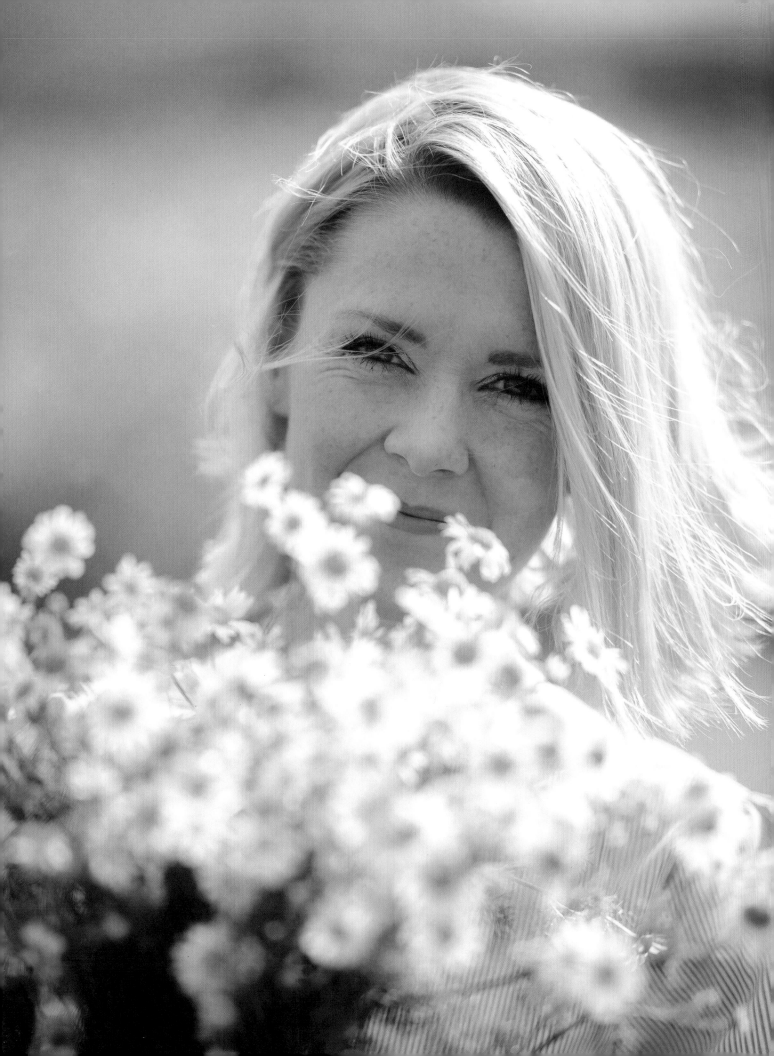

simply
sustainable
beauty

A collection of 50 simple zero waste beauty
recipes to give you naturally beautiful skin & hair

EMILIE WOODGER-SMITH
Photographs by Joab Woodger-Smith

WHITE OWL

To Mum, thank you for always encouraging me to believe.
What started with searching for fairies at the bottom of the garden
turned into real potion making and writing this book.
This is for you.

First published in Great Britain in 2021 by
PEN & SWORD WHITE OWL
An imprint of Pen & Sword Books Ltd
Yorkshire – Philadelphia

ISBN 9781526795182

Group Publisher: Jonathan Wright
Series Editor and Publishing Consultant: Katherine Raderecht
Art Director: Jane Toft
Editor: Katherine Raderecht
Photography: Joab Woodger-Smith

Printed and bound in India, by Replika Press Pvt. Ltd.

Pen & Sword Books Ltd incorporates the Imprints of Pen & Sword Books
Pen & Sword Books Limited incorporates the imprints of Atlas, Archaeology, Aviation,
Discovery, Family History, Fiction, History, Maritime, Military, Military Classics, Politics,
Select, Transport, True Crime, Air World, Frontline Publishing, Leo Cooper, Remember
When, Seaforth Publishing, The Praetorian Press, Wharncliffe Local History, Wharncliffe
Transport, Wharncliffe True Crime and White Owl.

For a complete list of Pen & Sword titles please contact:
PEN & SWORD BOOKS LIMITED
47 Church Street, Barnsley, South Yorkshire S70 2AS, England
E-mail: enquiries@pen-and-sword.co.uk
Website: www.pen-and-sword.co.uk
or
PEN AND SWORD BOOKS
1950 Lawrence Rd, Havertown, PA 19083, USA
E-mail: Uspen-and-sword@casematepublishers.com
Website: www.penandswordbooks.com

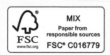

contents

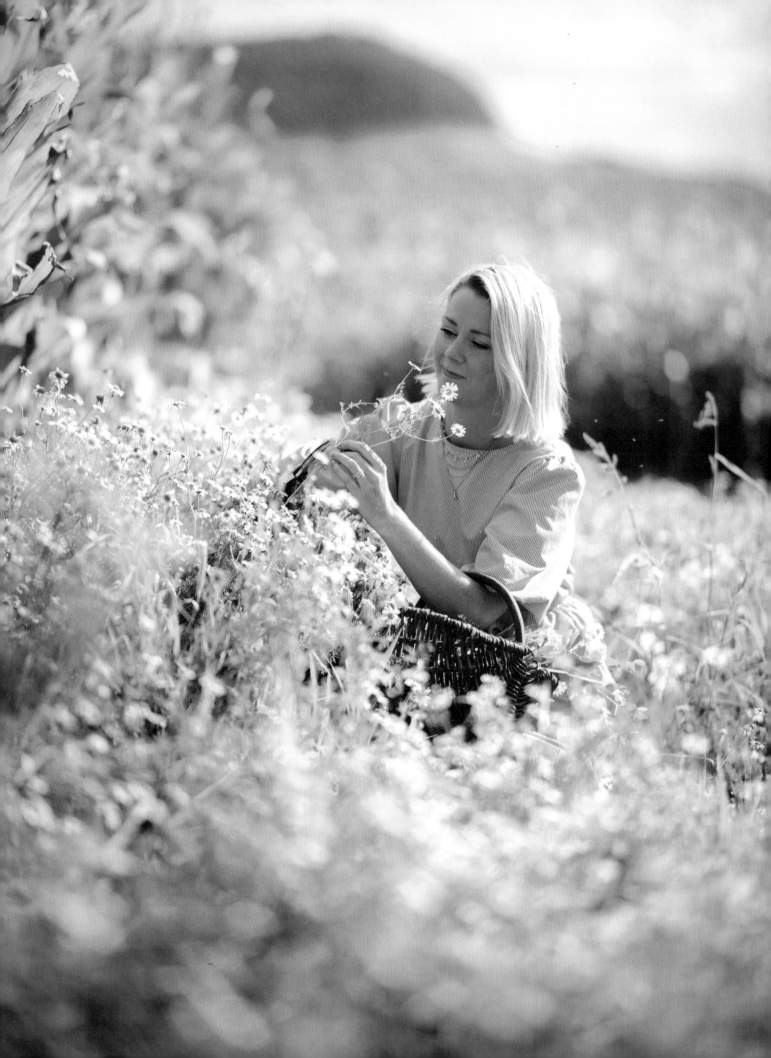

introduction

The beauty industry is often portrayed as being full of glitter and perfection, but the ugly side of the beauty industry is that it produces an astronomical amount of unnecessary waste.

About 120 billion units of packaging is mass produced by the beauty industry every year; much of it plastic. This translates to billions and billions of plastic bottles, tubs, pots, sprays and tubes making their way into our homes. In addition to the huge amount of plastic used to create packaging for beauty containers, approximately 18 million acres of woodland is deforested every year to produce the virgin paper and card used to display these products. Plastic containers are made of mixed materials and often have complex designs, which means they are very rarely able to be recycled. The plastic created by the beauty industry is destined to be used once before being disposed of and, very often, it finds its way into our beautiful oceans.

Single-use plastic waste is currently entering our oceans at a rate of around 11 million metric tons a year. It is harming marine life, damaging habitats and disrupting ecosystems. If we keep consuming at this rate, the amount of plastic in our oceans is set to triple by 2040. This will have a devastating effect on our marine ecosystems and wildlife.

The beauty industry makes huge amounts of money by persuading us to buy *more and more* products - most of them unnecessary. It is an industry that wants us to buy the latest products, the newest shades, the freshest scents. The message is just to buy and keep on buying. Nothing about the beauty industry system is sustainable. I don't believe we can continue in this way.

Okay! Enough of the scary stuff. What can we do about it? Because we have to do something, right?

I believe the best thing we can all do as individuals, is to slow down our rate of consumption and reduce the number of products we buy from these giant companies that are harming our planet. If enough of us stop buying products packaged in single-use plastic, the rate of production and consumption will slow, as will the impact on our planet.

"But Em, I don't want to turn into a smelly, dry skinned, lank haired hippy!", I hear you cry!

Fear not, there is another way to keep looking naturally beautiful, without having to buy into this planet-harming, mass consumerism. Learning how to make your own beauty products at home, personalised for you is how!

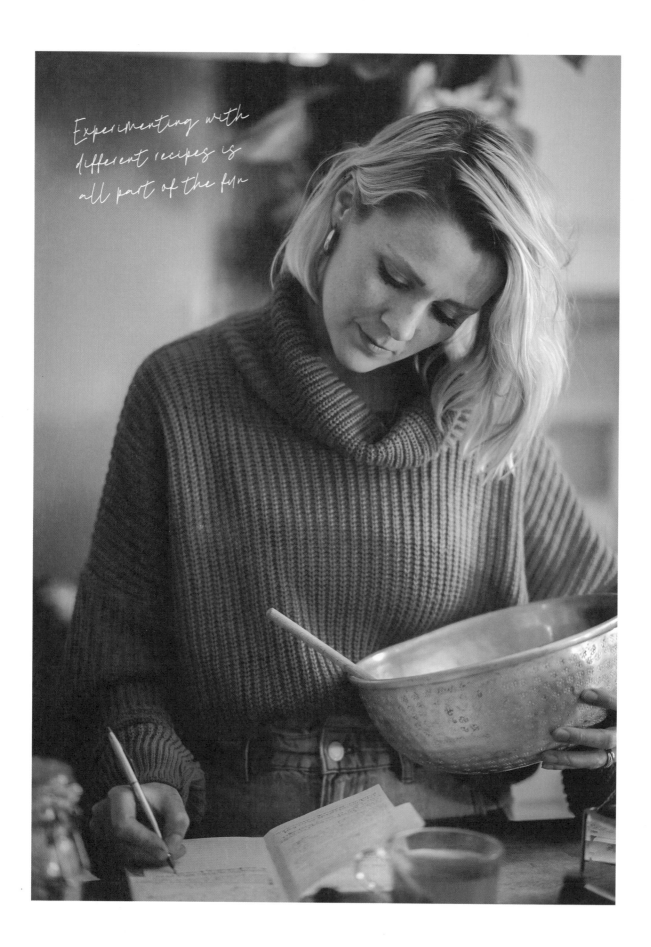

Experimenting with
different recipes is
all part of the fun

Throughout this book, I will show you exactly how to take care of your hair, body and skin without harming the planet by using simple, natural ingredients. I guarantee, you'll never go back to shop-bought beauty products after you've learned to make your own.

When you buy a beauty product you are very unlikely to know what it's made of, where the ingredients have come from or what impact those ingredients have had on the environment. You will also have no idea how much carbon was used in harvesting, refining, creating, packaging, shipping and transporting your products. There are so many hidden negative environmental factors behind that pretty new lotion bottle sitting on your bathroom shelf.

HOW DOES MAKING YOUR OWN PRODUCTS HELP?

Creating your own products, using sustainably sourced materials from producers that regenerate and care for habitats rather than destroy them, is a much more sustainable alternative to buying from the beauty industry giants. Buying the raw ingredients to make your own products at home cuts out all of the carbon heavy middle men.

When you make your own products, you can also use the same staple ingredients in so many recipes. This means you're only transporting those few raw products once, rather than several times for each product. Every time you make something of your own using your store cupboard ingredients at home, you're helping to reduce your waste and your environmental impact even further. You really only need a few natural ingredients to create all the products in your whole beauty and self-care routine.

THE BEST BIT

I found the best thing about making my own products is that they work so much better than the shop-bought ones I was using. I understand what different ingredients do and how to use them which means I can make products tailored specifically for my skin and hair. My skin is softer, less patchy and clearer; I have fewer breakouts, my hair is healthier and even my armpits are less sweaty and definitely not smelly!

This book will teach you how to create your own skin care routine using only the best (sustainably sourced, of course) natural ingredients. You'll find you don't need the 101 lotions and potions you've been told you must buy to have naturally, beautiful skin and you will reduce your environmental impact at the same time.

I'm so excited to be sharing these recipes with you and hope they spark the same love of making your own beauty products as they did for me. Happy making!

Please note that the recipes in this book do not guarantee results and should not be used to treat any kind of medical condition. Please consult a medical professional before trying these recipes if you have a skin condition or allergy.

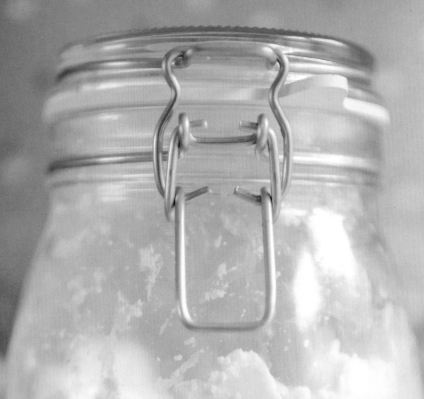

ingredients

To make most of the recipes in this book you only need a few staple ingredients. You'll be amazed at how easy to get hold of and versatile these ingredients are.

When it comes to buying ingredients, try to buy Soil Association approved organic, cruelty free products and, where possible, Fair Trade. I will always try my local zero waste shop first before searching online and you should too, if you're lucky enough to have one nearby. Every little helps when it comes to reducing your impact on the environment.

I try to buy direct when shopping online to avoid using the corporate giants like Amazon. There is a list of my go-to suppliers in the Supplier Directory at the end of the book.

PLASTIC PACKAGING

Where possible try to choose ingredients that are completely naked or packaged plastic-free. Some ingredients may only be available in plastic packaging, but it's still much better for the environment to get Fair Trade, organic, natural ingredients that are packaged in plastic that you can reuse at home or dispose of responsibly, compared to buying a non-sustainably sourced product that's packaged plastic-free.

STAPLE INGREDIENTS

1. Cocoa Butter – Solid at room temperature and made from cocoa beans, this rich butter smells like vanilla and chocolate - divine. When used in skin care, cocoa butter moisturises your skin and creates a barrier, protecting it from environmental damage. Cocoa butter works really well in body butter, to help to keep your skin moisturised and smelling fantastic.

2. Shea Butter – Soft, silky and rich in fatty acids, antioxidants and vitamins A & E, this butter is so fantastically good for your skin I use it in nearly all of my skin care creams. It is very soothing so it's perfect for skin conditions like eczema.

3. Coconut Oil – This is a light oil, semi-solid at room temperature that easily melts into your skin. It's naturally antibacterial, smells gorgeous and I use in most of my recipes.

4. Sweet Almond Oil – This is the perfect light carrier oil for skin and hair care products. Sweet almond oil contains high amounts of vitamin E & A which improves the appearance of your skin. It is quickly absorbed, helping to even out your skin tone and lift dark marks.

5. Aloe Vera Gel – Calming and cooling, aloe vera gel comes from the fleshy insides of the Aloe plant. It's perfect for treating burns and can help repair damaged skin. It's also great in hair care products; it moisturises and defines curls, adding bounce and shine.

6. Beeswax – Naturally antibacterial and a by-product of honey production, I use beeswax in many of my skin care recipes. Beeswax forms a protective layer on your skin, and attracts moisture from the air, helping to keep your skin hydrated.

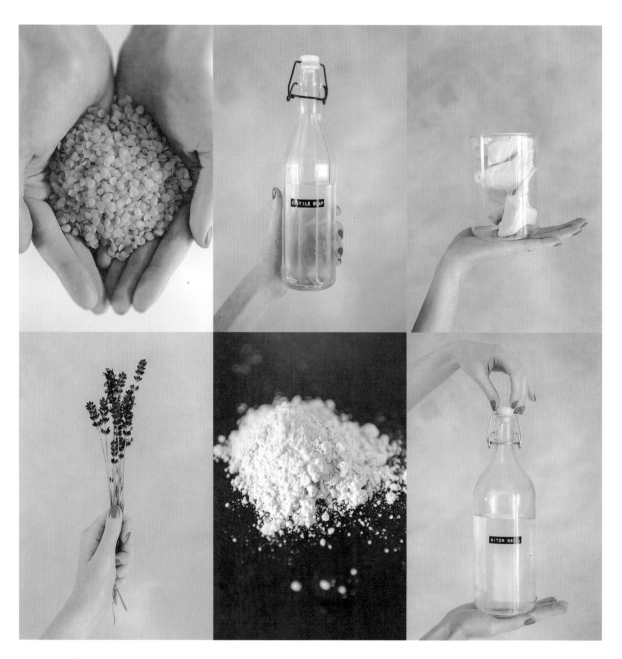

Beautiful natural ingredients Clockwise from top left, **BEESWAX** a wonderful by-product of honey production **CASTILE LIQUID SOAP** a super-concentrated natural plant based soap **COCOA BUTTER** rich buttery and smelling of vanilla and chocolate **WITCH HAZEL** a natural astringent from the branches and twigs of the Witch Hazel shrub **KAOLIN CLAY** a naturally occurring clay which makes a great exfoliator **LAVENDER** a bushy strong-scented plant from the Mediterranean commonly used in aromatherapy.

Clays – When used in skin products clay can act as a brilliant exfoliator, removing dead skin cells. When allowed to dry out on the skin, clays draw out impurities and toxins from the pores so they are perfect for face masks.

- **Bentonite clay** – This clay is derived from volcanic ash and is negatively charged which means it must not come into contact with metal or it will become toxic! Always use wooden or plastic spoons when using this clay. Bentonite clay is brilliant for using in skin and hair care for its detoxifying properties.
- **Kaolin Clay** – A great natural exfoliator, this clay adds texture to homemade beauty products. It can help to soothe irritated skin, reduce excess oil and brighten and tone your skin. It can even be used as a dry powder shampoo; just dust over your hair and roots, leave to sit and then rinse out.
- **Pink French Clay** – Wonderful for your skin, this clay contains high levels of iron oxide which encourages skin cell renewal, leaving it looking healthier and brighter. Pink French clay is perfect for using on mature and damaged skin, just add water to make a paste and use as a face mask once a week to reduce the appearance of wrinkles.

Vitamin E – This is the nectar of the gods when it comes to skin care! Vitamin E oil has incredible anti-ageing and skin protecting properties. A little goes a long way.

Olive Oil – An extra rich and nourishing oil for your skin, it is full of antioxidants and vitamin E. Olive oil is brilliant for your hair and works perfectly in a hair mask.

Apple Cider Vinegar – Using raw, organic apple cider vinegar has amazing benefits for your hair. It helps to balance the pH of your scalp and flattens the cuticles of your hair making it super silky, shiny and tangle free. It also helps to remove product build-up that can leave your hair feeling lank and greasy.

Coloured powders (beetroot, cranberry etc) – Vegetables, fruit & flowers that have been dehydrated and ground down into a powder are a great alternative to chemical pigments when it comes to natural makeup.

Soap Nuts – Not really nuts, these are actually the dried berries from a tree native to Nepal. They contain natural saponins when soaked in hot water. Saponins lift dirt, grease and grime and are perfect for using as a natural cleaning agent for your skin and hair. They also make a great homemade laundry liquid.

Distilled Water – This is simply water that has been brought to the boil and left to cool. The boiling process kills off unwanted bacteria. You can use it to extend the shelf life of homemade products without the need for preservatives.

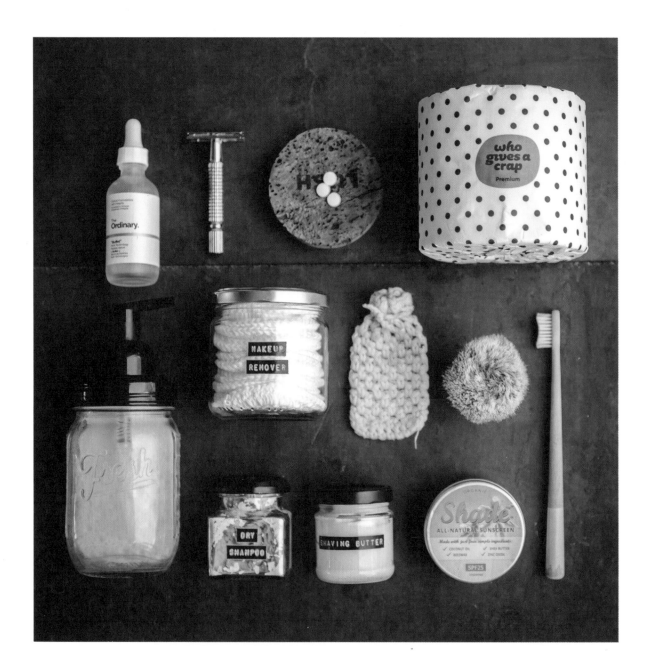

Some of my favourite products Clockwise from top left, **BUFFET** from The Ordinary is a favourite serum from this sustainable brand **REUSABLE RAZOR** from Mutiny **LOO ROLL** with no plastic from Who Gives A Crap **NAKED TOOTHBRUSH TABLETS** from Dentab **SUN CREAM** with no plastics from Shade **SHAVING BUTTER, DRY SHAMPOO, HAND SOAP** and **MAKEUP REMOVER** all homemade **SOAP SAVER POUCH** made from reusable 100% cotton crochet rounds and old **MAKEUP BRUSH** for dry shampoo.

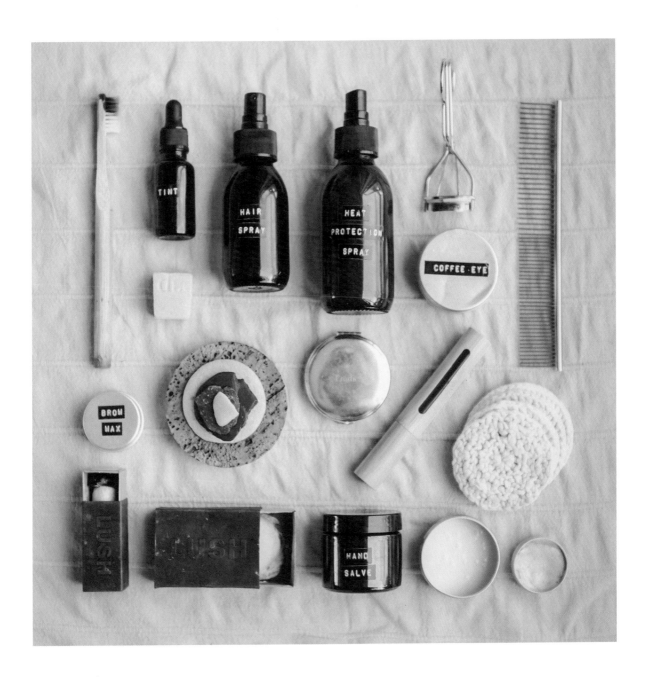

Head to toe beauty products Clockwise from top left, **BAMBOO TOOTHBRUSH**, **SOAP SLICE**, DIY **NAIL OIL**, **HAIRSPRAY**, **HEAT PROTECTION SPRAY** and **COFFEE EYE BALM**, metal **EYELASH CURLERS** and **COMB**, reusable **COTTON ROUNDS**, DIY **SHIMMER BLUSH**, **DEODORANT**, **HAND SALVE**, plastic-free **FOUNDATION** and **HIGHLIGHTER STICK**, DIY **BROW WAX**, solid bars of **SHAMPOO**, **CONDITIONER** and **FACE PRIMER**, metal Links London **MIRROR**, plastic-free **MASCARA**.

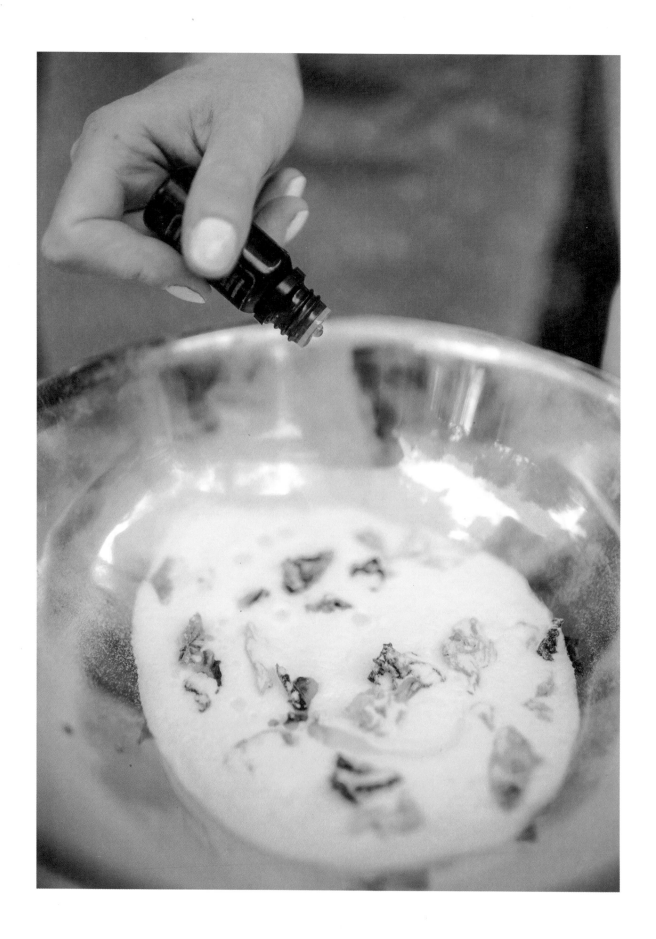

essential oils

I love to use essential oils in my homemade beauty products for their beautiful scents and botanical properties. They really help to enhance and personalise the products. Often essential oils are the star of the show; the recipe just wouldn't work without them. Essential oils can help to improve your skin's elasticity and appearance, fight bacteria, tighten pores, calm irritation and even invigorate blood flow to encourage cell renewal and quicken the healing process. They really are magic in a tiny bottle.

WHAT ARE ESSENTIAL OILS MADE OF?
When you peel an orange or crush a mint leaf, you get an explosion of scent. This is because as you tear and crush plants you are breaking their cells, releasing the natural oils. It is that natural oil which is extracted to create a plant essential oil. Essential oils are super concentrated, meaning you only need a few drops to get the benefits and beautiful scent of the plant. Extracted oils have very small molecules, which means they can penetrate through our skin, nourishing much more deeply than any other oil or cream ever could. Essential oils can really enhance your homemade beauty recipes, improving the appearance of your skin whilst adding a beautiful scent.

HOW DO YOU USE OILS?
You can add a few drops of essential oils into your creams, oils, powders and baths to perfume them. I've suggested particular essential oils for each recipe, but if you want to experiment, swap them out for an oil that works for you and your skin.

MY TOP SIX BEAUTY ESSENTIAL OILS
Lavender – By far my favourite essential oil, I love the scent of lavender, which takes me straight back to summer holidays in the South of France, but I also love the affect it has on my skin. Lavender has calming qualities that soothe dry and itchy skin; its antibacterial properties help to heal cuts and scrapes and reduce breakouts on your skin. The scent of lavender is calming and I love to add a few drops to a bath or in my diffuser as I'm heading off to sleep.

Frankincense – This is the golden essential oil when it comes to skin care. Frankincense has the ability to minimise wrinkles, tone skin, tighten pores and even out your skin tone, reducing the appearance of sun damage and breakouts. It has a woody scent which adds a touch of luxury to your homemade beauty products. It's a scent that would cost a lot of money in shop-bought products. I always include this oil in my face serums for its brilliant qualities.

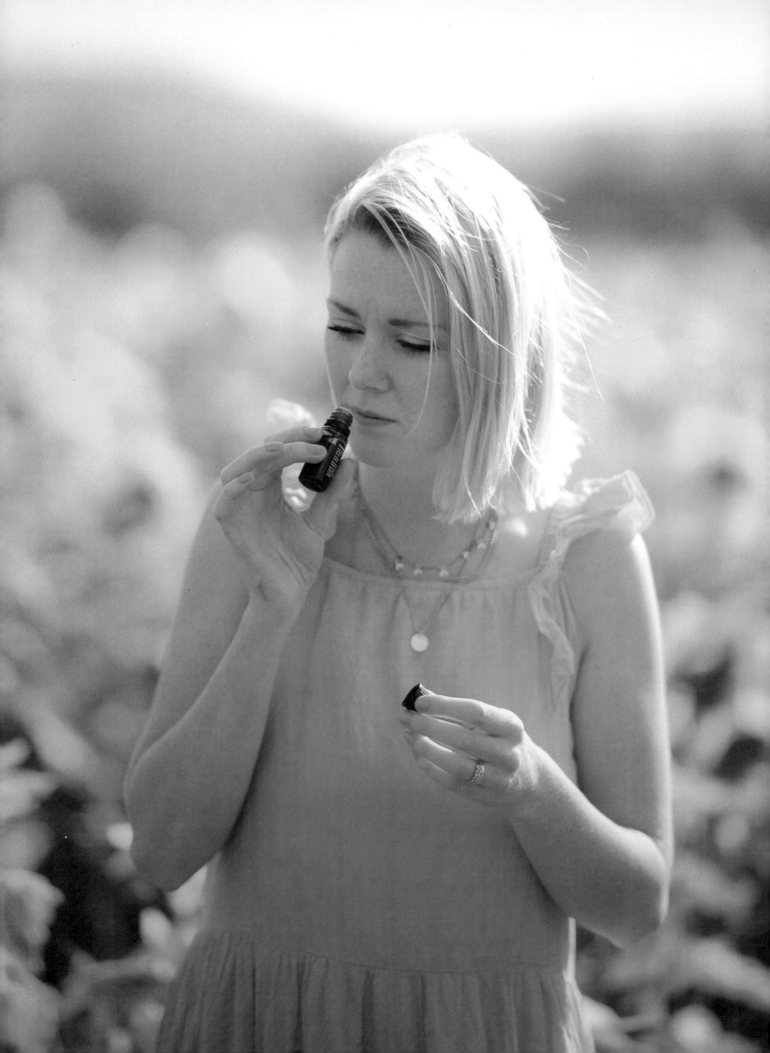

Rose – One of the oldest essential oils, rose oil has been used for centuries in skincare all over the world. It has the ability to heal and rejuvenate your skin. Rose oil is also brilliant for using on stretch marks to reduce their appearance or on skin damage where it can help to repair the skin. Rose oil also has mild antiseptic qualities which make it great for using in your facial skin care routine to help prevent breakouts.

Orange – Possibly the most uplifting and refreshing of the essential oils, orange is always a good idea in my book. Smelling exactly like a freshly peeled orange, this oil encourages your skin to create more collagen, revitalising your skin to leave it looking brighter and clearer. Orange oil is brilliant for using on oily skin types to leave your skin looking dewy and fresh. I love to use this oil in my morning beauty routine because its scent really wakes me up and makes me feel fresh as a daisy.

Rosemary – This is the best essential oil for using in your homemade hair products. It helps to boost circulation when applied to the scalp, stimulating the hair follicles, increasing hair growth and reducing hair loss. Rosemary also helps to reduce the chance of a dry scalp and dandruff. Its cleansing qualities make your hair shiny and healthy so is perfect for your hair products.

Eucalyptus – This oil reminds me of lazy spa days and I love having it in my skincare routine. It has mild antiseptic qualities that make it perfect for using on your face. Eucalyptus will help to reduce the chance of breakouts and heal broken skin, reducing reddening. It's also a great skin toner, helping to keep on top of oily, combination and acne prone skin. I love to use eucalyptus oil in the shower in the morning; a few drops in the corner of the shower tray will leave your morning shower feeling like a spa steam treatment.

When it comes to buying your essential oils, make sure you research the companies you are buying your oils from. The industry is currently unregulated and you want to make sure you know what's in that little bottle before putting it on your skin. I've included a list of my preferred suppliers that sell essential oils in the Supplier Directory at the back of the book.

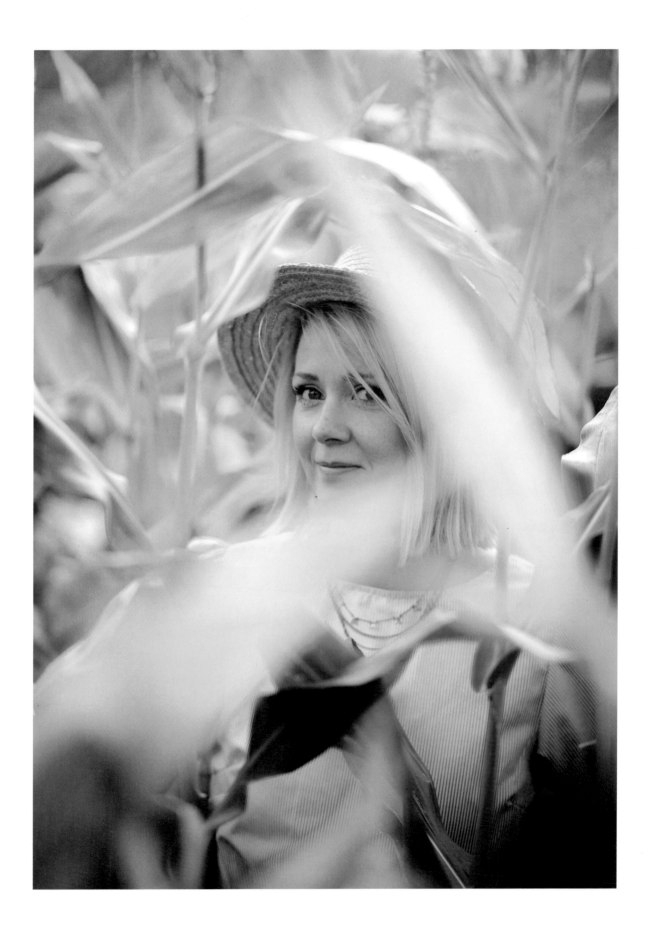

knowing your skin type

As I've already mentioned, one of the best things about making your own beauty products is that you can really personalise them to your own skin and scent preferences.

I don't know anyone that has been born with perfect, flawless skin. We all seem to fall into one of three skin types; dry, oily or combination skin. All these skin types require different products to keep them looking radiant and healthy.

If you're not sure what kind of skin you have, here are the characteristics of the three main types and how to treat them:-

Dry skin

This skin type is unable to retain much moisture which leads to dry flaky skin. The lack of moisture means fine lines and wrinkles are easily formed. Skin pores are small due to the lack of natural oil production from the skin.

Dry skin requires more external nourishment than other skin types. Using salves, creams and moisturising ingredients like shea butter are perfect for keeping dry skin moisturised. Using a water based toner spritz can help to keep skin hydrated throughout the day. Avoid using anything that might strip away the small amount of natural oil that your skin produces. It's best to steer clear of synthetic foaming soaps and alcohol based toners as they will dry your skin.

I find that lavender oil is brilliant for dry skin. It has calming qualities which help to soothe and heal dry, irritated skin.

Oily skin

Large pores, blackheads and breakouts are common characteristics of this skin type. Most people go through an oily skin phase during their teenage years when breakouts are much more common. Oily skin tends to look a little shiny or greasy because of the over-production of oil by the skin.

Oily skin loves clay, it helps to absorb excess oil without stripping your skin. Avoid synthetic foaming agents that strip your skin of oil. They make your skin's oil glands over produce oil, leaving your skin greasy - the opposite of the desired effect. Using oils to clean oily skin is ideal; oils mix together and when rinsed off with a hot cloth, remove your skin's excess oil and clear out your pores without stripping your skin. A light face oil like jojoba oil is great for oily skin, but you only need to use a tiny amount.

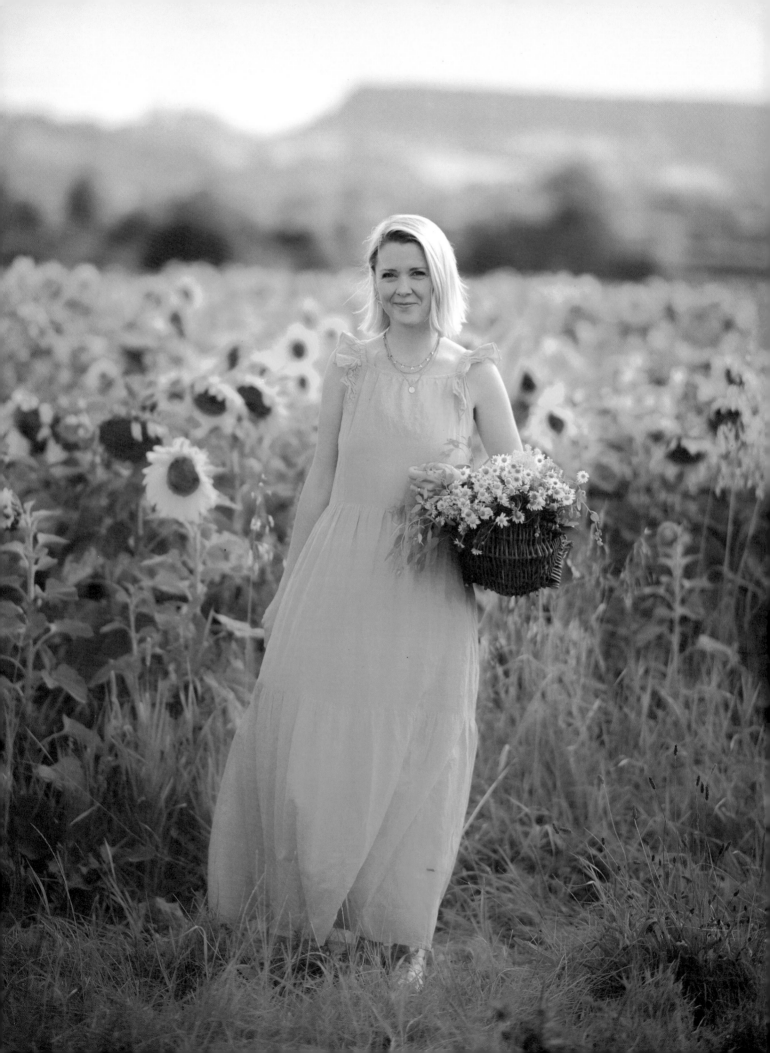

Citrus oils like grapefruit and orange are fantastic for oily skin as they are great degreasers and can help to clarify oily skin and clean out clogged pores.

Combination skin
This is a very common skin type, where people have both dry and oily areas in their skin. The most common oily area is the T-zone - the area around the nose, chin and forehead. Dry patches can form around the eyes and edges of the face.

Combination skin is the hardest skin type to manage as you have got to try and treat two contrasting skin types. I think working on the two areas separately is the best way to manage this skin type. To cleanse combination skin, use a light oil and a hot cloth wash as it works as well for both oily and dry skin.

Geranium essential oil is great for balancing your skin and is perfect on combination skin.

Knowing how to manage your skin type is the key to having a great skin care routine.

SIMPLY SUSTAINABLE BEAUTY

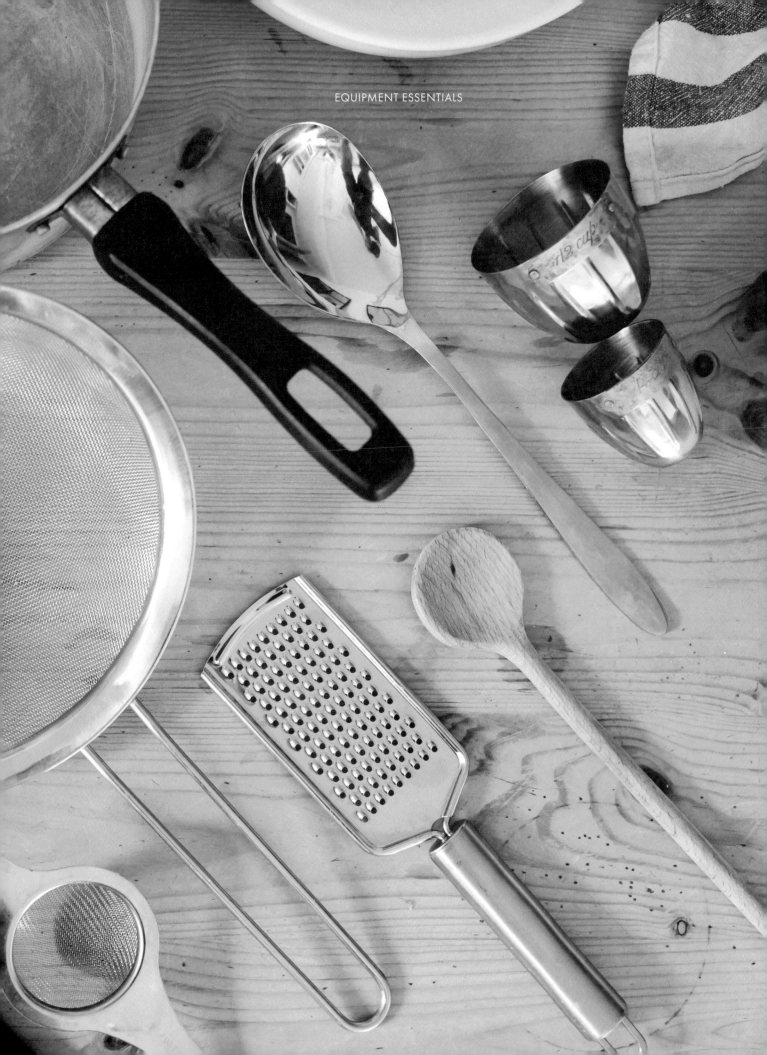

equipment essentials

To make the products in this book you won't need to go out and buy a load of new equipment. You're likely to already own everything you need and, if not, they are all easily found in charity shops or second hand online.

Most of the equipment you need can be used for both food and beauty recipes with a good hot soapy clean in between. The only items I would keep purely for beauty recipes are a wooden spoon and a spatula as you can never truly get rid of the essential oil scents and no one wants eucalyptus flavoured scrambled eggs!

CONTAINERS

When it comes to containers, I am all for reuse and upcycling. If you have a favourite glass bottle or jar, wash it out, stick a ribbon on it and you're good to go! Don't discard jars when you've finished with the product either; just keep washing and reusing them much as you can.

Keep an eye out for coloured glass containers as these are perfect for preserving the natural properties of essential oils. You can keep products in clear glass, but they will need to be kept out of the light.

Plastic is not a great option when it comes to containers. Plastic tends to soak up scents which means smells can get muddled when they are refilled. You are also unable to store the essential oils used in my recipes safely in plastic containers, as

the oils will break the plastic down. It's best to stick to glass or metal containers.

MEASURING

I measure out all my recipes in cups, spoons and drops. This makes it much easier to measure your ingredients and means you don't require weighing scales. You can buy a cup measuring set from most hardware and cooking stores. A spoon measuring set is vital for this book; you will find they are easy to find online or on your local high street.

DOUBLE BOILER

When it comes to melting down ingredients I always try to use a double boiler. A double boiler is a large non-plastic bowl resting over a pan of boiling water. It is nothing fancy and does the job well. I'd recommend keeping a bowl specifically for your beauty DIYs to avoid getting beeswax in your next cake.

LABELLING

There are many plastic-free ways you can label your beauty products. Some blackboard paint and a piece of chalk works really well, although paper stickers, or just a marker pen are great too.

Controversially, I do use a plastic label maker. I use my label maker because the labels last and last. You can wash them over and over and the lettering doesn't budge, or start to look a bit sad round the edges. Switching to homemade beauty products is a long term solution for me, so I want a labelling system that's here for the long haul. Plus, my handwriting is terrible!

NEED TO KNOW

Before we dive into making our own products, there are a few pieces of general advice to share with you.

Keeping clean

Make sure you have washed and dried your hands to remove any bacteria that could get into your products during making. Hot soapy water will do nicely.

Make sure all your equipment and containers are also sparkling clean before you start. Running everything through the dishwasher on a hot wash is perfect, or a good soapy hand wash and dry in a warm oven works well too.

Your work space

Ensure your work space is clear and you have everything you need to hand. When you're working with waxes and butters that set quickly, you don't want to suddenly realise you can't find your spatula!

The clean up

When you've finished creating and it's time for the clean-up, don't be tempted to pop everything in the dishwasher. The waxes, butters and oils will block your machine and it is very difficult to get it working well again after that. Yes, I am speaking from first-hand experience!

The best way to clean up is to reheat the bowl and equipment, wipe away as much as you can with kitchen roll to absorb the excess oils nicely. Once you've got off as much product as possible, give your equipment a hot soapy wash and buff dry with a tea towel. You can pop the kitchen roll into your compost bin to break down happily, without blocking any drains!

Water

You need to avoid getting any non-distilled water into any of the products in this book. This is because water can create mould and bacteria.

Water based products need preservatives to keep them shelf stable, otherwise the water goes off and will ruin your product within a few days.

For this reason, I only ever use distilled water for my recipes, never tap water. Check out the ingredients section for how to make your own distilled water.

Storage & Shelf Life

As you're making natural products without preservatives, there will be a differences in how long each product will last, depending on their ingredients.

Butter, wax and oil based products will last the longest time; around 6 to 9 months and sometimes even longer. Let your nose be the judge when it gets past 6 months after being made.

Products that are made with distilled water will last much less time; 1 to 3 months if kept in a cool dark place.

Products with fresh ingredients will need to be used virtually straight away. I will always let you know when this is the case in each recipe.

Now, let's get started.

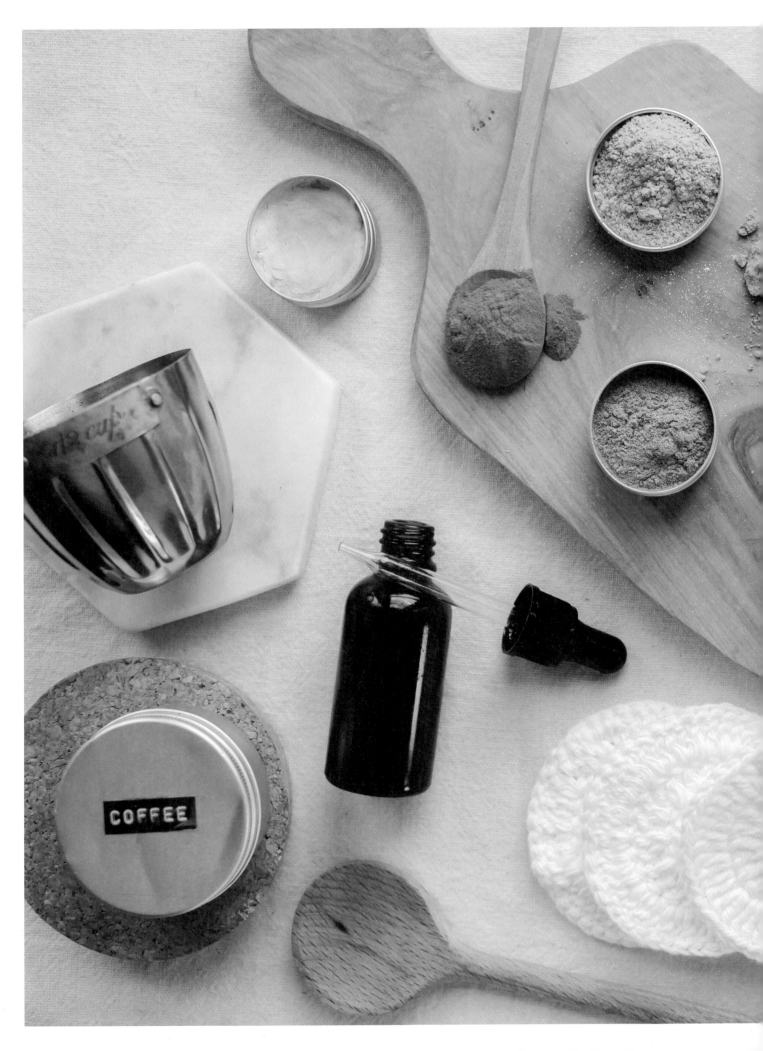

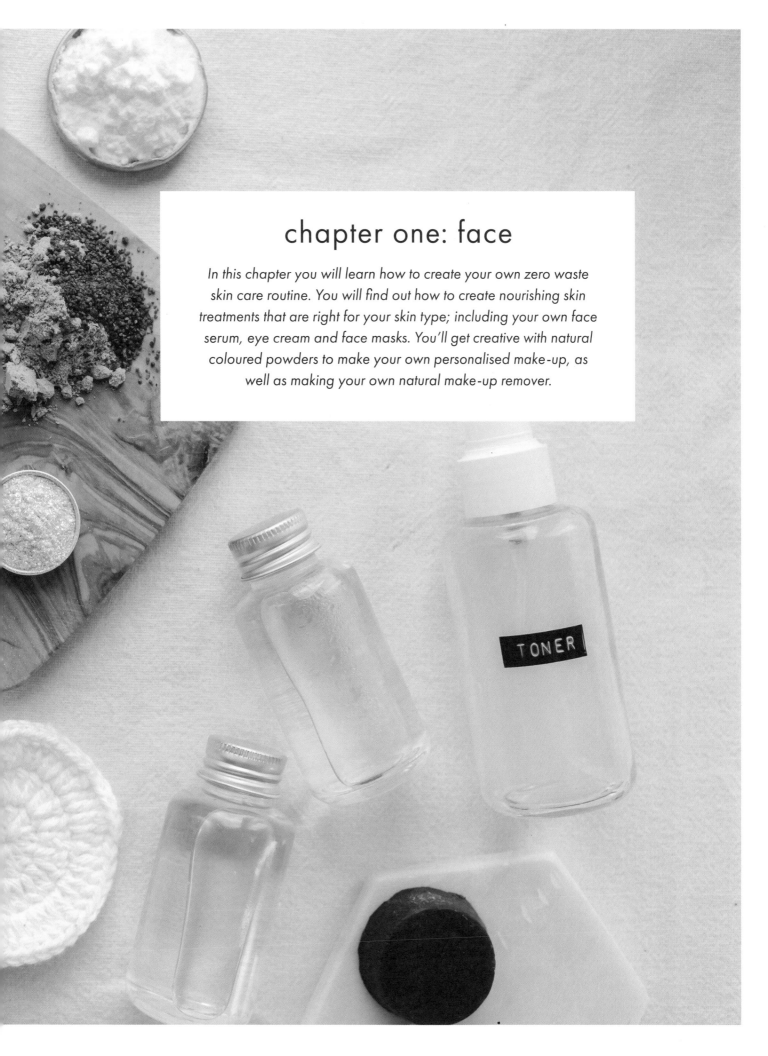

chapter one: face

In this chapter you will learn how to create your own zero waste skin care routine. You will find out how to create nourishing skin treatments that are right for your skin type; including your own face serum, eye cream and face masks. You'll get creative with natural coloured powders to make your own personalised make-up, as well as making your own natural make-up remover.

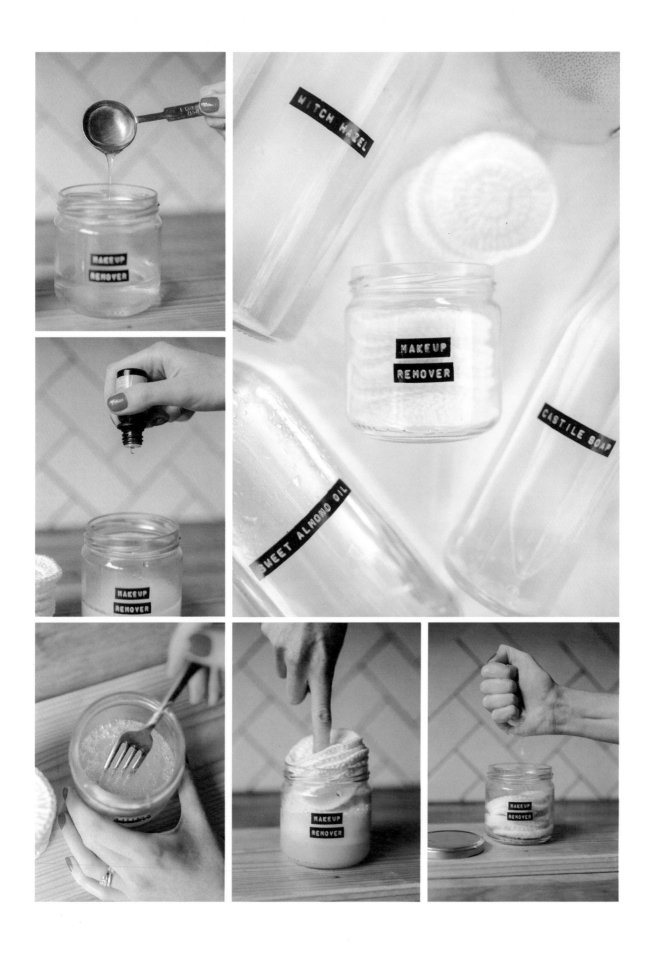

eucalyptus & grapefruit cleansing wipes

If you are the kind of person who uses wet wipes to remove your make-up person (like I used to be), this is a fantastic zero waste swap. You can remove your make-up and cleanse your skin quickly and easily. Even if you don't wear make-up, this is a great cleansing solution for anyone.

What you'll need

- 6 tbsp Distilled water
- 1 tbsp Witch hazel
- 2 tbsp Sweet almond oil
- 1 tbsp Castile Soap
- Essential oils
  3 drops of Eucalyptus
  3 drops of Grapefruit
- Make-up cleansing pads
  I recommend 100%
  cotton rounds

HOW TO MAKE

1. Pour all the ingredients into a reusable container and whisk to combine.

2. Carefully place your cleansing pads into the same container and push them down firmly into the bottom.

3. Seal your container and tip it upside down to ensure all the cleansing pads are covered in the solution.

4. Leave for 5 minutes to make sure all the cleansing pads are fully saturated.

5. You can either tip out the excess water to have slightly moist cleansing wipes, or leave the liquid in and just squeeze the excess off each time you use them for more of a wet wipe.

6. They are ready to use!

Emilie's tips

- If you buy 100% organic cotton cleaning pads they will last you for years and can go on the compost heap when that time comes. They can be rinsed immediately after use then scrubbed with soap and water to clean. Leave them in the sun to dry as the UV rays will bleach out any stains.

- This cleansing liquid will keep for up to one month in a cool place out of direct sunlight.

- Use different oils to suit your skin type. Rose is good for combination skin, Sandalwood for dry skin and Geranium for oilier skins.

- I use an old coconut oil jar for this recipe. It is the perfect size for round cleansing pads.

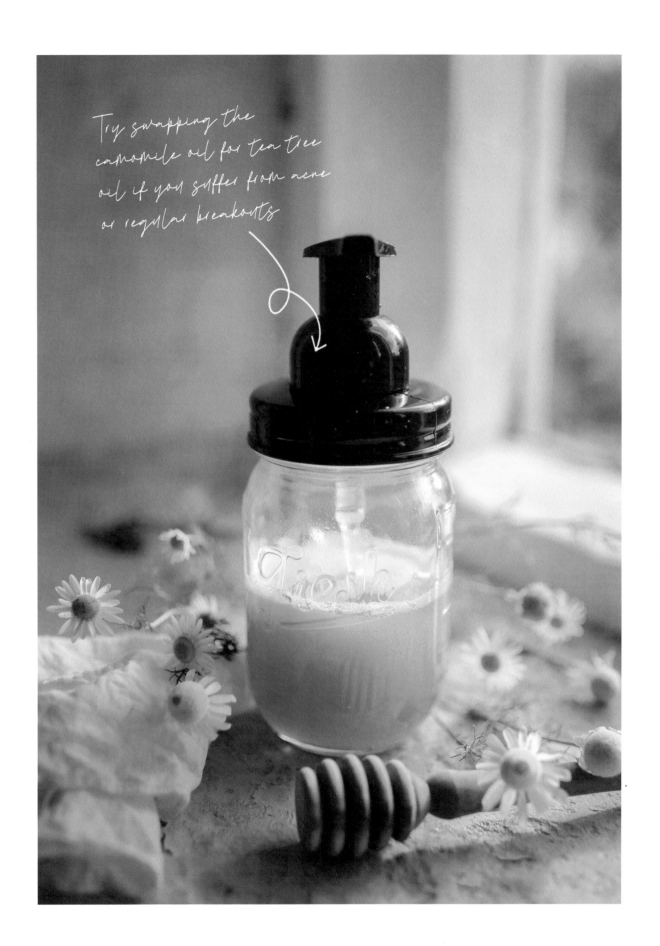

Try swapping the camomile oil for tea tree oil if you suffer from acne or regular breakouts

cleansing honey face wash

This face wash is a naturally calming and hydrating face cleanser. It's great for sensitive and dry skin as it contains honey to keep your skin from drying out. It is also antibacterial and will help prevent breakouts.

What you'll need

- 5 tbsp Runny honey (preferably raw & local)
- 4 tbsp Castile soap
- 3 tbsp Distilled water
- 1 tsp Sweet almond oil
- 2 drops Camomile essential oil

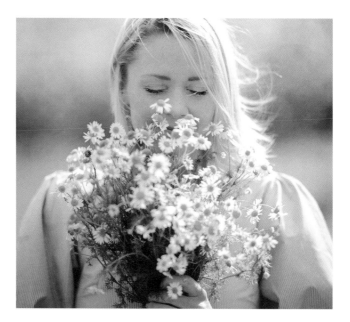

HOW TO MAKE

1. Measure out the oil, honey and soap into your soap dispenser container.

2. Add in the essential oils and swirl to combine.

3. Top up with distilled water and, using a fork, whisk all the ingredients together.

4. Pop the lid on and you're ready to go!

Emilie's tips

- Most camomile essential oil is made in the UK. Look out for local suppliers to reduce your environmental impact.
- This oil has amazing calming qualities for your skin and is perfect for using on sensitive skin.
- Buy a foaming pump bottle to get the most from this soap.

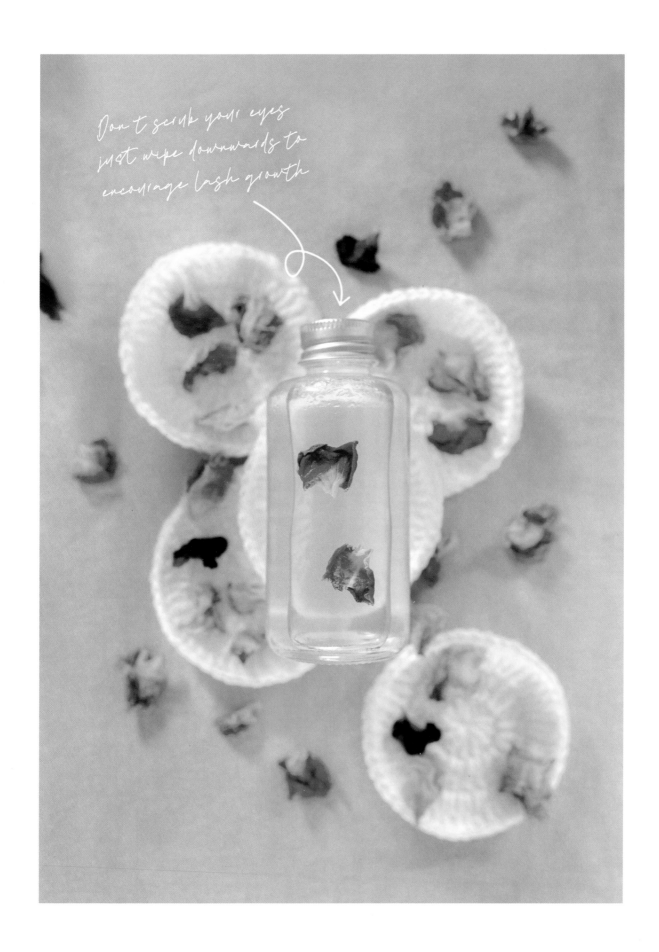

Don't scrub your eyes just wipe downwards to encourage lash growth

floral micellar water

Yes, you really can make your own 'magic water' at home, using natural plant based oils and scents; it's so much better for your skin than commercial petroleum based micellar waters. This DIY will leave your skin feeling moisturised and super clean. It does a great job of gently removing eye make-up and cleansing your skin of all the dirt and pollution that can build up throughout the day.

What you'll need

- ■ 6 tbsp Distilled water
- ■ 2 tsp Witch hazel
- ■ 1 tsp Glycerine – plant based
- ■ ½ tsp Sweet almond oil
- ■ 2 drops of Rose geranium essential oil

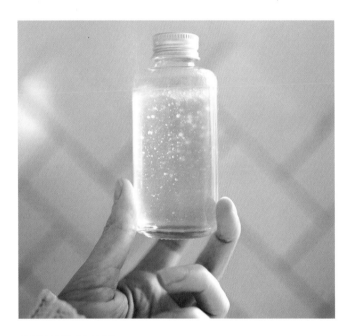

HOW TO MAKE

1. Measure all your ingredients (except for the essential oil) out into a jug and whisk with a fork to combine.

2. Pour your mixture into your clean bottle.

3. Drop the essential oils directly into the bottle and shake to combine.

Emilie's tips

- ■ I use my water on reusable make-up remover cotton pads and swipe over my eyes to remove my eye make-up.

- ■ This will keep for around one month so only make as much as you'll need each time.

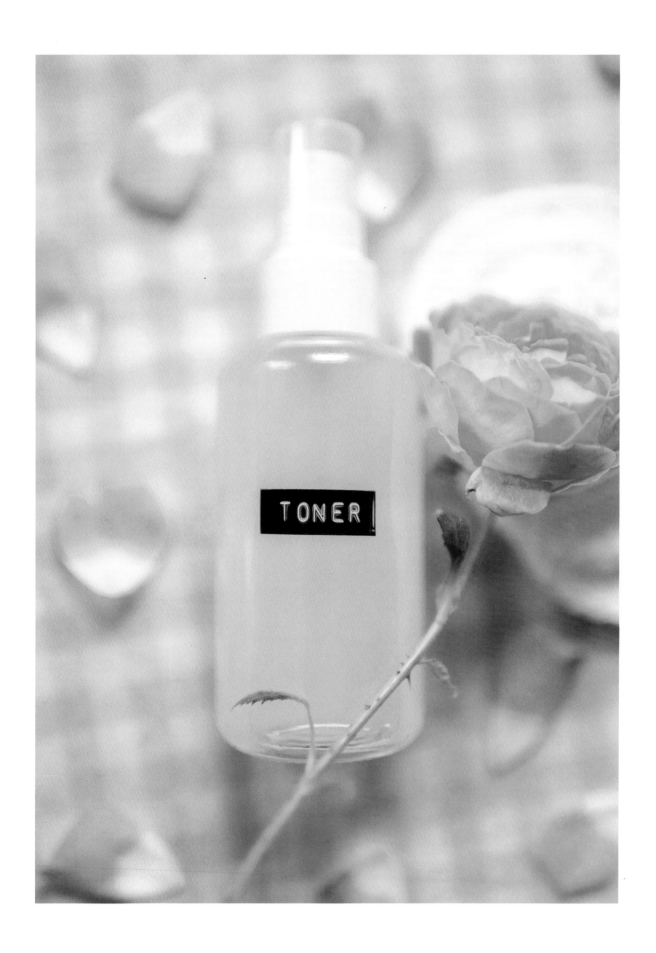

frankincense & rose toner

This nourishing and soothing skin toner is perfect for using after washing your face to help restore the skin's natural oils. This recipe uses rose and frankincense essential oils which have fantastic anti-ageing properties; they improve skin elasticity and reduce the appearance of fine lines.

What you'll need

- 2 tbsp Aloe vera gel
- 2 tbsp Witch hazel
- ¼ tsp Vitamin E
- 3 tbsp Distilled water
- 4 drops Frankincense essential oil
- 3 drops Rose essential oil

HOW TO MAKE

1. Pour all the ingredients into a bottle and shake thoroughly to combine.

2. Top up with distilled water.

3. That's it – you're done!

Emilie's tips

- You can use this toner in an atomiser spray bottle or by pouring a small amount onto a reusable cotton pad or scrap of fabric and dabbing your face after washing and before applying serums.

- Vitamin E is the miracle ingredient in this recipe. It's a natural antioxidant and protects your skin from the pollutants and free radicals that can cause skin damage.

- On hot days this is a fantastic cooling facial spritz. It's also great for using when you've just come out of the sea and need a refreshing boost.

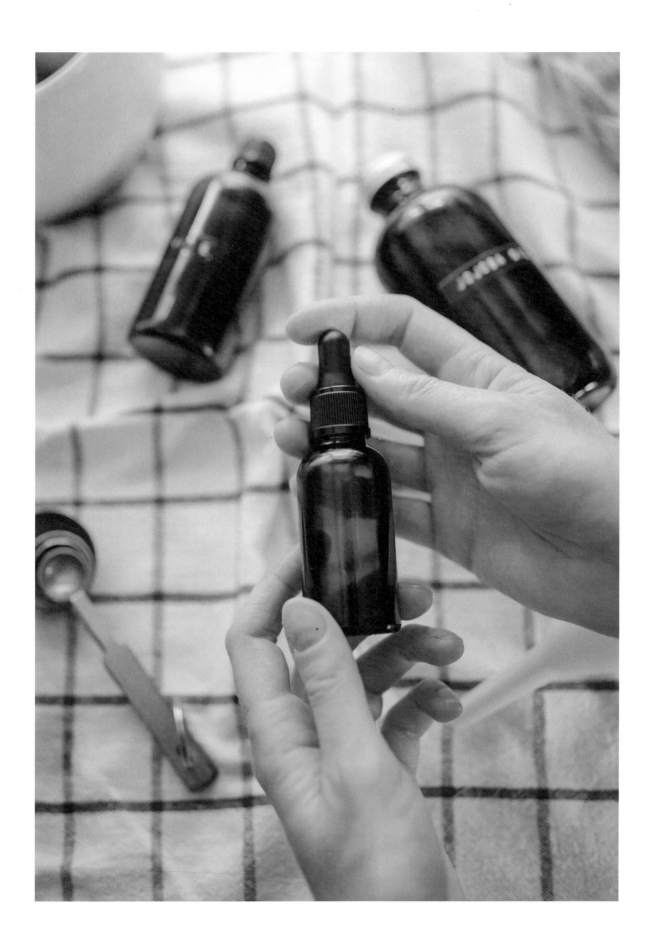

anti-ageing face serum

Are you still buying lotions and potions that claim to be the next wonder skin product, but seeing no difference except an ever growing pile of single-use plastic? After you've tried this face serum you'll know you've found that wonder product you're after with the bonus of no single use plastic packaging or a hefty price tag. Packed with vitamins, antioxidants and rejuvenating essential oils, this face serum is the bee's knees!

What you'll need

- 2 tbsp Sweet almond oil
- ½ tsp Vitamin E
- 1 tbsp Jojoba oil
- 5 drops Frankincense essential oil
- 2 drops Carrot seed essential oil

HOW TO MAKE

1. Find a small bottle you love. A dropper bottle is perfect if you have one.

2. Measure out the oils and pour directly into the bottle, using a funnel if you needed.

3. Shake to combine.

Emilie's tips

- Use daily, morning and night. A few drops is all you need.
- Turn this into a calming night oil by adding a drop or two of lavender essential oil before massaging in.

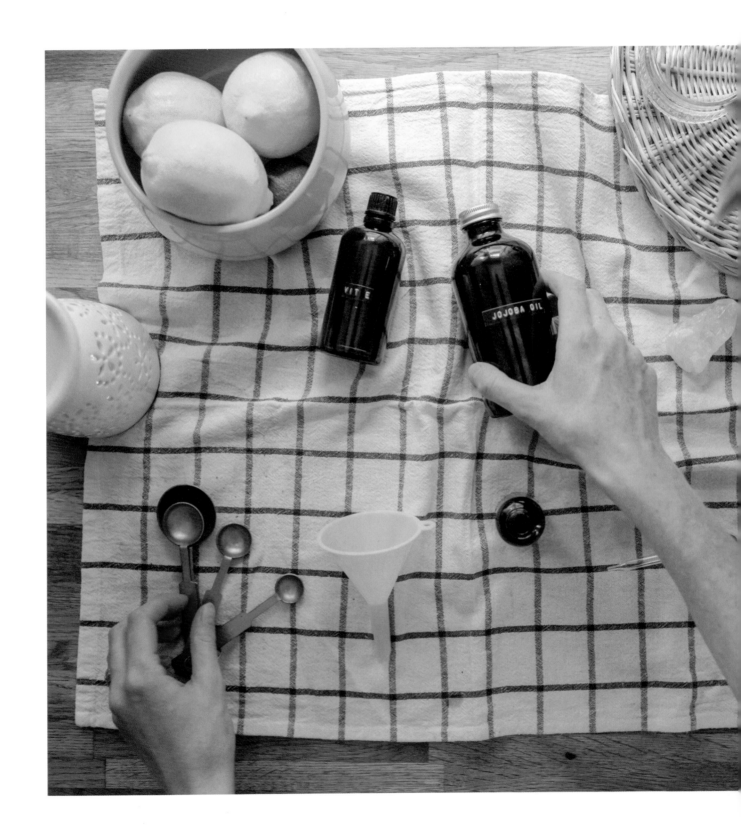

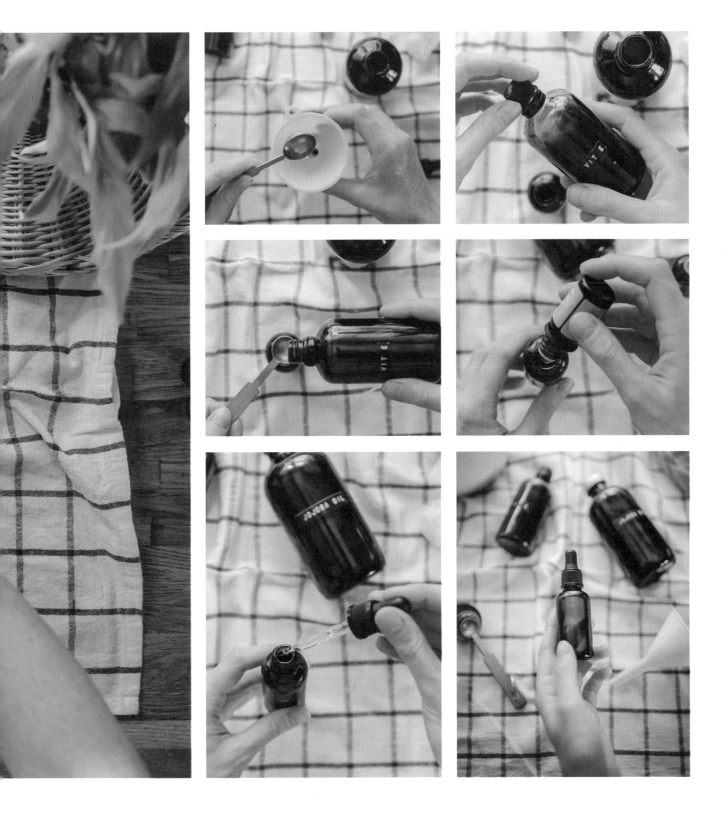

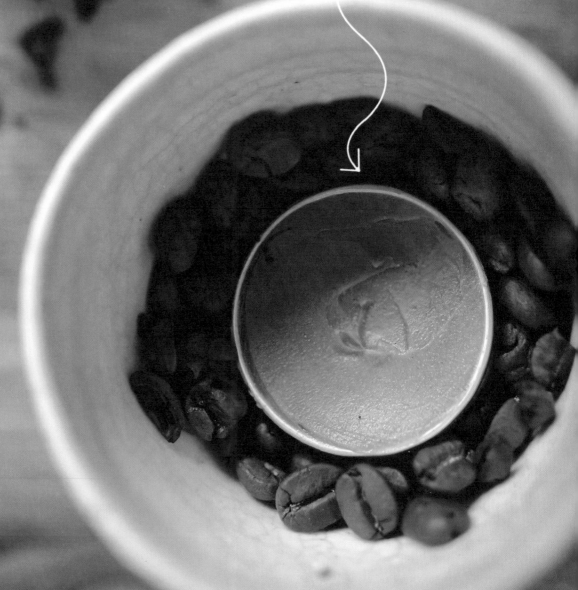

The sweet almond oil in
this eye balm can help
to lighten any dark
shadows under the eyes

morning coffee eye balm

This fresh coffee-infused eye balm gives your skin a boost of energy as the caffeine is absorbed into your bloodstream. It works best when used in the morning, helping to reduce puffiness and the appearance of dark circles. The antioxidants in the coffee beans also combat free radical skin cells that can prematurely age your skin. What more could you ask for from an eye balm?

What you'll need

For the infused coffee oil

- 1 tbsp Fresh coffee grounds
- 2 tbsp Sweet almond oil

For the balm
- 2 tsp Cocoa butter
- 1 tbsp Soya wax
- 2 tbsp Infused coffee oil

HOW TO MAKE
Infused Coffee Oil

1. Measure out the fresh coffee grounds into a clean glass jar with a lid.

2. Add in the sweet almond oil and shake to combine.

3. Seal the jar and leave the coffee to infuse with the oil on a sunny windowsill for around a week.

4. After the coffee has infused the oil will be rich and dark.

5. Strain the oil through a sieve and dispose of the grounds in your compost bin.

Eye Balm

1. Melt the soya wax and cocoa butter in a bowl over a pan of hot water.

2. When melted, take off the heat and add in your infused coffee oil.

3. Mix well until it is completely combined.

4. Pour the balm into your container.

Emilie's tips

- If you want to make the infused oil in a hurry, pop the open jar into a shallow pan of hot, but not boiling, water and leave for an hour to infuse.
- Swap coffee for Jojoba oil and add 4 drops of your preferred essential oil.

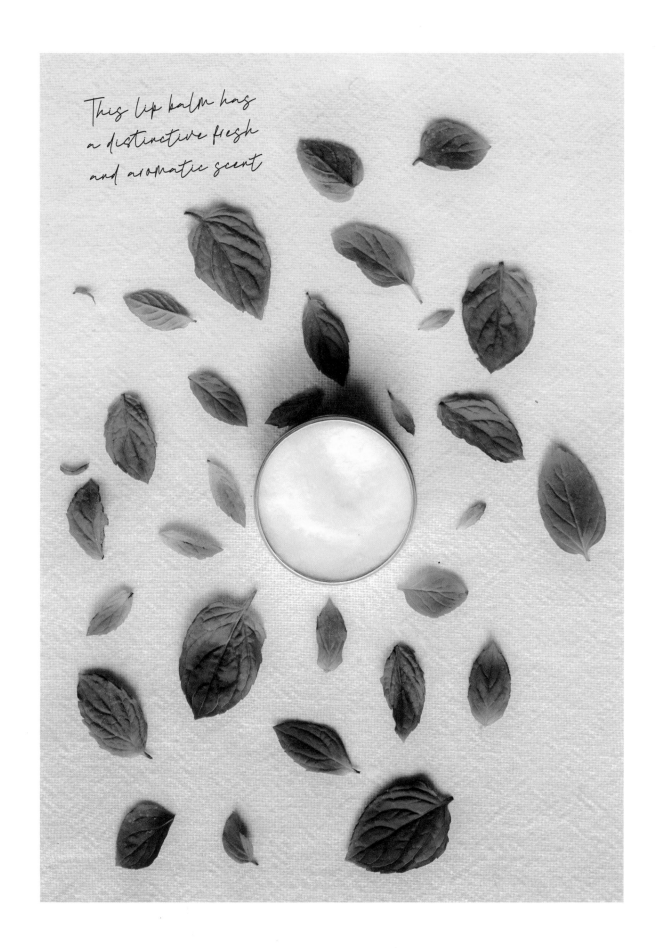

This lip balm has
a distinctive fresh
and aromatic scent

peppermint lip balm

This tinglingly minty lip balm is your best friend in the winter months. The shea butter and coconut oil keep your lips nourished and moisturised, while the soya wax creates a matt barrier to protect your lips against the elements. The peppermint essential oil creates the tingling sensation, bringing blood to the surface of your lips. This helps to heal any cracks and keep them soft and supple whatever the weather.

What you'll need

- ½ tsp Shea butter
- 2 tsp Coconut oil
- 1 tsp Soya wax
- 7 drops Peppermint essential oil

HOW TO MAKE

1. Measure out the shea butter, soya wax and coconut oil into an old glass jar.

2. Pop the glass jar into a pan of hot water and wait for the contents to melt.

3. Once melted, carefully remove the jar from the pan and leave to cool for two minutes.

4. Add the peppermint essential oil to the mixture.

5. Pour the mixture into your lip balm tin, pop the lid on and leave to cool overnight. You can speed this process up by putting it in the fridge for an hour.

Emilie's tips

- For a different scent variation, swap the peppermint oil for 3 drops of cinnamon, 2 drops of clove and 2 drops ginger and add in a pinch of cinnamon for a speckled finish. I call this Spicy Chia lip balm.

- Coconut oil will melt when you touch it so if you want a portable version, reduce the amount of coconut oil and increase the amount of soy wax. The balm won't melt when you pop it in your back pocket.

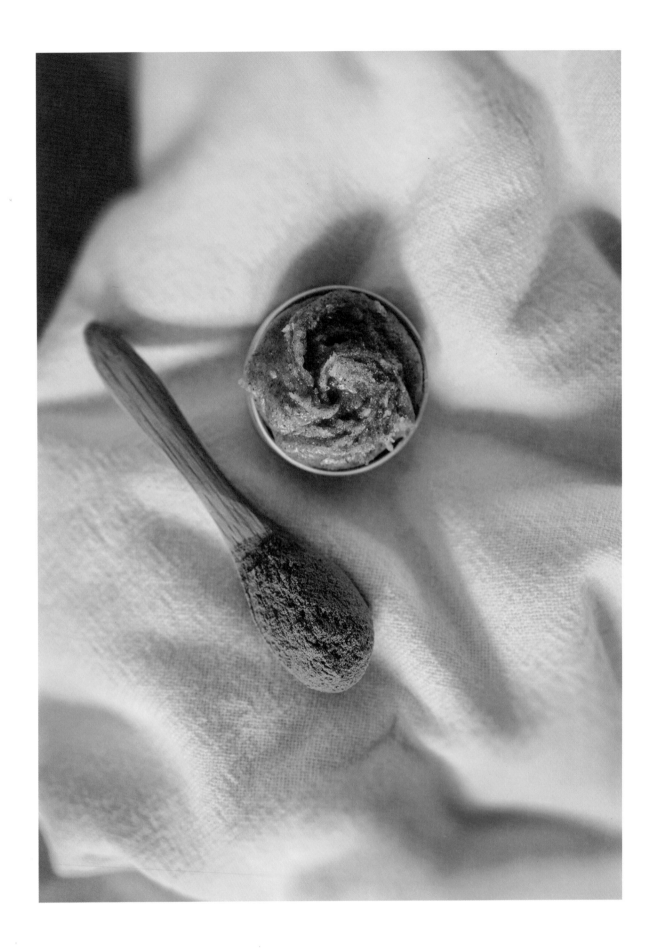

plumping cinnamon lip scrub

Lip scrubs are a great way to keep you lips supple during the winter months, when central heating and harsh weather can dry them out. This scrub uses spices to help pump blood to your lips which makes them look plumper and feel rejuvenated.

What you'll need

■ 1 tsp Coconut oil

■ 1 tsp Caster sugar

■ ¼ tsp Ground cinnamon

■ A pinch of ground ginger and clove

HOW TO MAKE

1. Measure out the coconut oil and sugar into a bowl and combine using a fork.

2. Pop in the cinnamon and other spices and mix until distributed evenly.

3. Scoop the lip scrub into a cooled, sterilised tin and seal.

HOW TO USE

Use by placing a small amount on your lips and then rub them together. The sugar will act as an exfoliant, leaving your lips super smooth.

Emilie's tips

■ When your lips feel all tingly and soft, I love to lick off the remaining scrub for a zero waste sweet treat.

■ Mix up the spices in this recipe to your taste. A ginger spiced scrub is one of my favourites.

■ Spices naturally plump up your lips by increasing the blood flow.

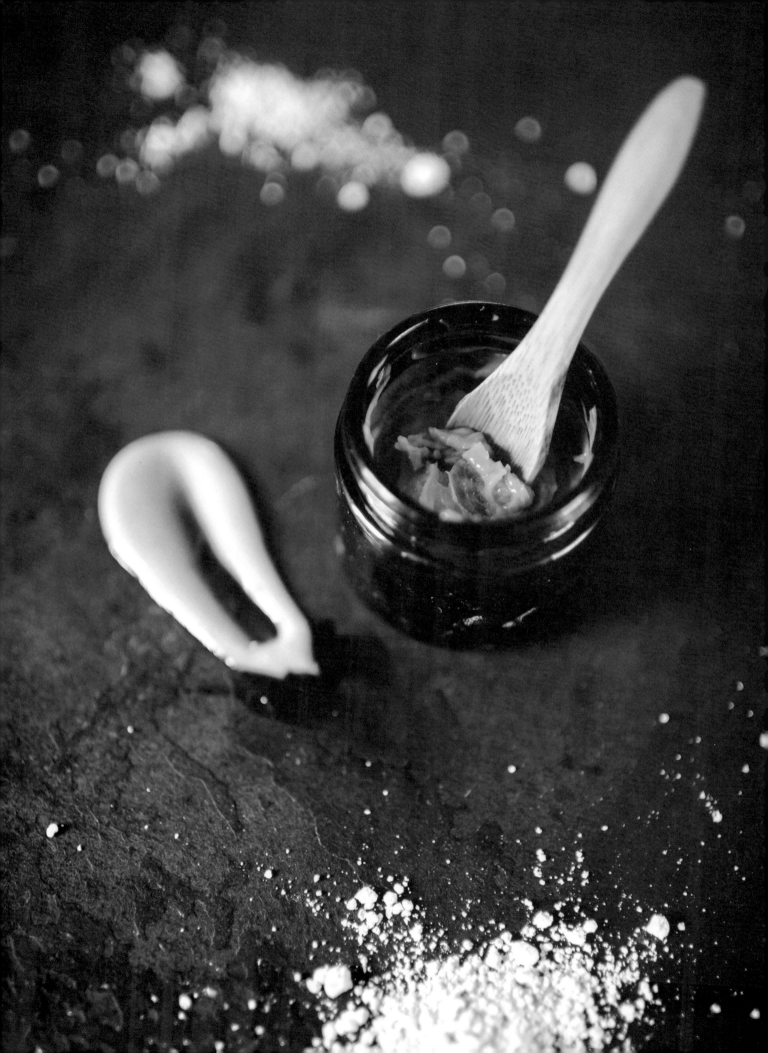

clay cleansing balm

This DIY clay cleansing balm is a firm staple in my nighttime skincare routine. It leaves my skin clean, make-up free and silky soft. The oil in this recipe breaks down your make-up (even waterproof mascara) with ease, the orange essential oil clears out the grease in your pores and the clay draws out impurities in your skin. The dream combination.

What you'll need

- 1 tbsp Sweet almond oil
- 2 tbsp Jojoba oil
- 1 tbsp Coconut oil
- 1 tsp Beeswax
- 2 tbsp Bentonite clay
- 1 tbsp Bicarbonate of soda
- 6 drops Orange essential oil

HOW TO MAKE

1. Put a non-metallic bowl over a pan of boiling water and add the beeswax and coconut oil. Stir with a wooden spoon until melted.

2. Take off the heat and add in the sweet almond and jojoba oils, stirring to keep any lumps from forming.

3. Add the bentonite clay using a wooden spoon (do not use a metal spoon as contact with metal turns bentonite clay toxic which can damage your skin) and bicarbonate of soda and stir until completely combined.

4. Add the essential oil and stir again before decanting into your chosen container.

Emilie's tips

- Don't use anything metal during this DIY as it will react with the bentonite clay, denaturing some of its properties.

- I apply this balm with a wooden lollipop stick directly to my dry skin and massage it in. I steam it off with a hot muslin cloth, splash with warm water and pat my skin dry.

- If you don't have bentonite clay, swap for pink French clay or kaolin clay instead.

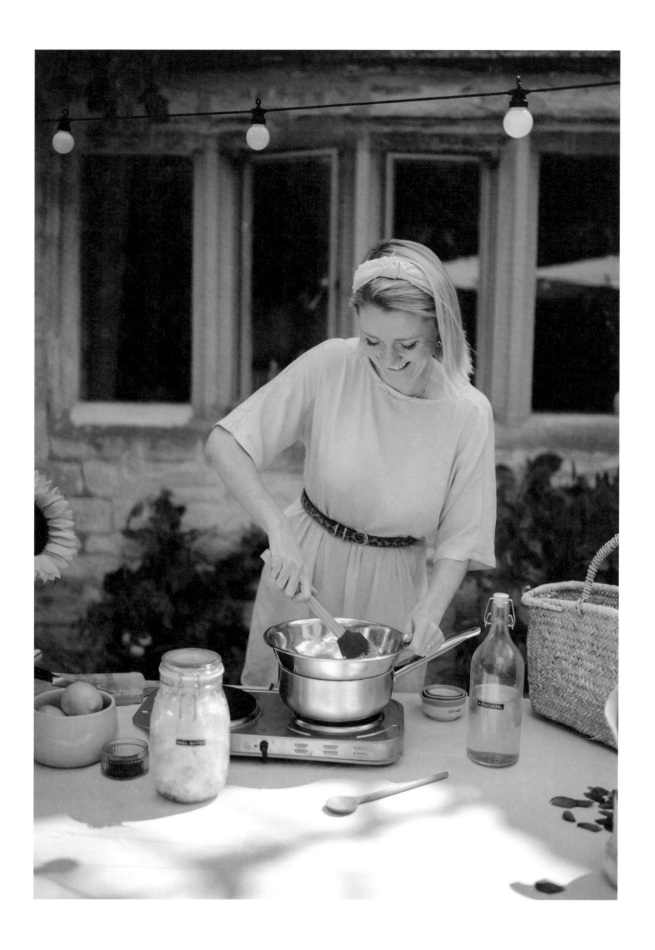

activated charcoal face wash bar

These face wash bars are a great addition to your zero waste travel toiletry kit. Perfect for travelling as they are completely solid, they are packed with ingredients to help prevent breakouts and clear out your pores.

What you'll need

- 3 tsp Activated charcoal powder

- 200g Shea butter & oatmeal soap base

- 1 tbsp Witch hazel

Essential oils

Tea Tree (antibacterial and helps prevent spots), *Frankincense* (evens skin tone and improves elasticity) *Lemon* (helps to cut through oil and grease, cleaning out your pores).

- 10 drops Tea tree essential oil

- 5 drops Frankincense essential oil

- 5 drops Lemon essential oil

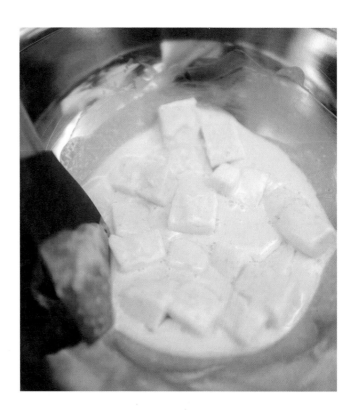

Emilie's tips

- Try and keep your bar dry in between uses to extend its shelf life. If you haven't got a draining soap dish, a great zero waste DIY is to criss-cross two elastic bands or hair bobbles over a jam jar lid and pop your bar on top!

- If you are using a non-silicon mould, you will need to wipe over the inside of the cases with a light oil (such as sunflower) and line them with a strip of baking paper to help you lift out the bars from the moulds.

- A great zero waste trick is to use a milk or juice carton cut in half as a mould. Once turned out, slice into soaps.

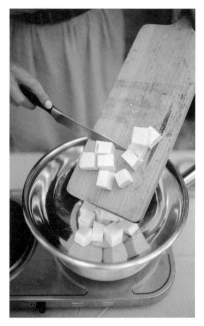

1. Cut the soap base into cubes and put into a heat-safe bowl.

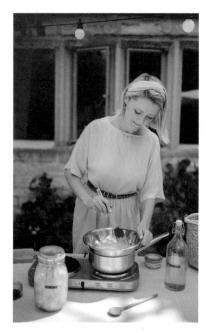

2. Put the bowl over a pan of boiling water and stir the soap cubes until they have melted.

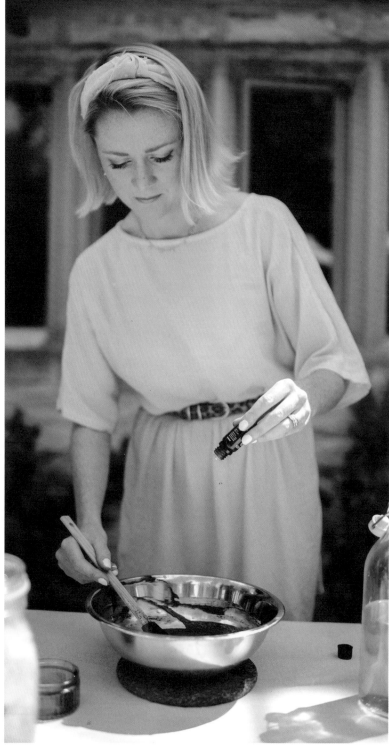

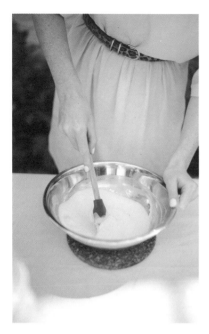

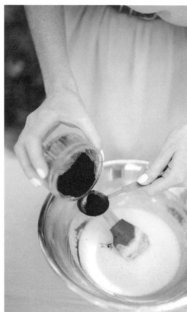

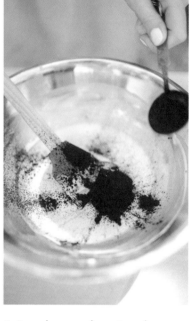

3. Take off the heat and add in the activated charcoal, witch hazel and essential oils, stirring until they are all fully combined.

4. Pour the soap base into the mould and leave to set for 2 hours.

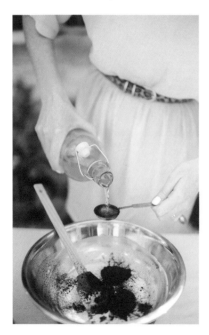

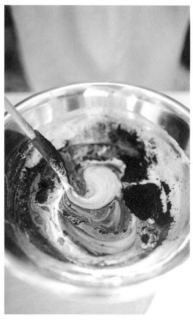

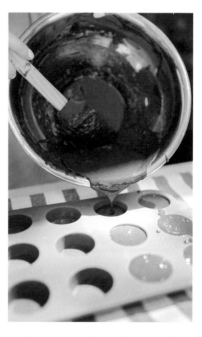

5. If you're using a metal tray, put in the freezer for the last 20 minutes to help you remove from the mould.

6. Once set, pop your soaps out of the moulds and leave to cure overnight in a cool place.

7. The soaps will then be ready for you to use in your morning face cleansing routine!

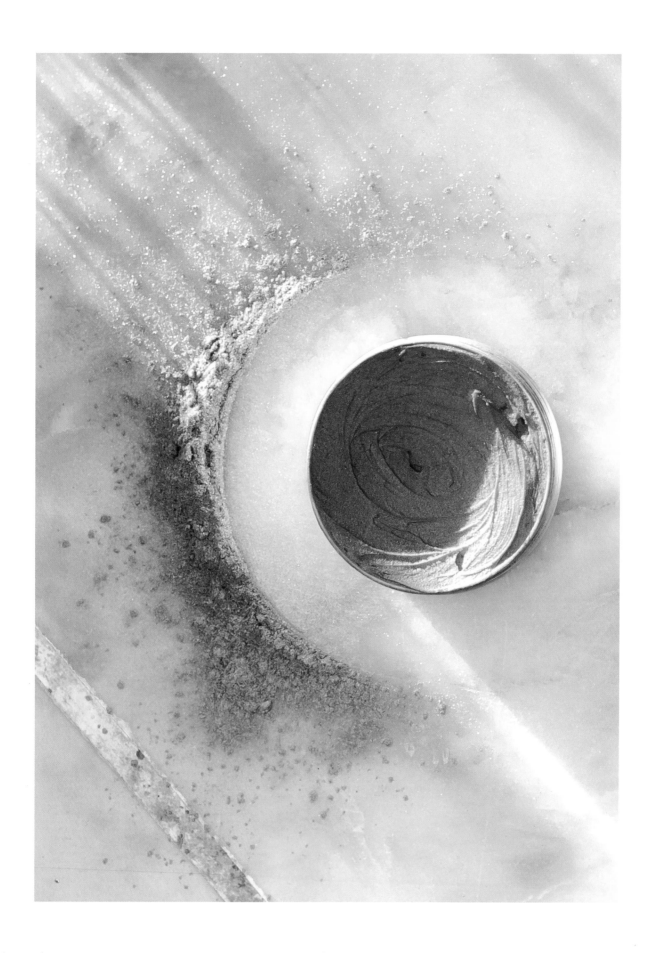

shimmer highlighter cream

Most shop bought highlighters use micro plastics to give them shine. These particles pollute our waterways and oceans when we wash our make-up off in the sink. This highlighter cream is made using synthetic mica powders which are completely plastic free and compostable. Think of it as letting you have your sparkly cake and eating it too!

What you'll need

- ½ tsp Pink mica powder
- 1 tbsp Sweet almond oil
- 2 tsp Soya wax
- ¼ tsp Cornflour

HOW TO MAKE

1. Melt the wax and sweet almond oil together in a bowl over a pan of water. When completely melted, take the pan off the heat.

2. Add in your chosen mica powder and cornflour and mix until fully combined.

3. Keep mixing until the ingredients begins to bind together. This will ensure your shimmer powder is evenly distributed throughout the cream.

4. Transfer the cream into a small tin or jar and leave to completely set for half an hour or so.

5. Your cream is now ready to use!

Emilie's tips

- You can customise your highlighter colour by changing the colour of the mica powder pigments to suit your skin tone.
- I love the pink and silver shimmer of this recipe, but add a bronze mica for a more golden glow in the summer or go silver for a cool highlight in the winter.

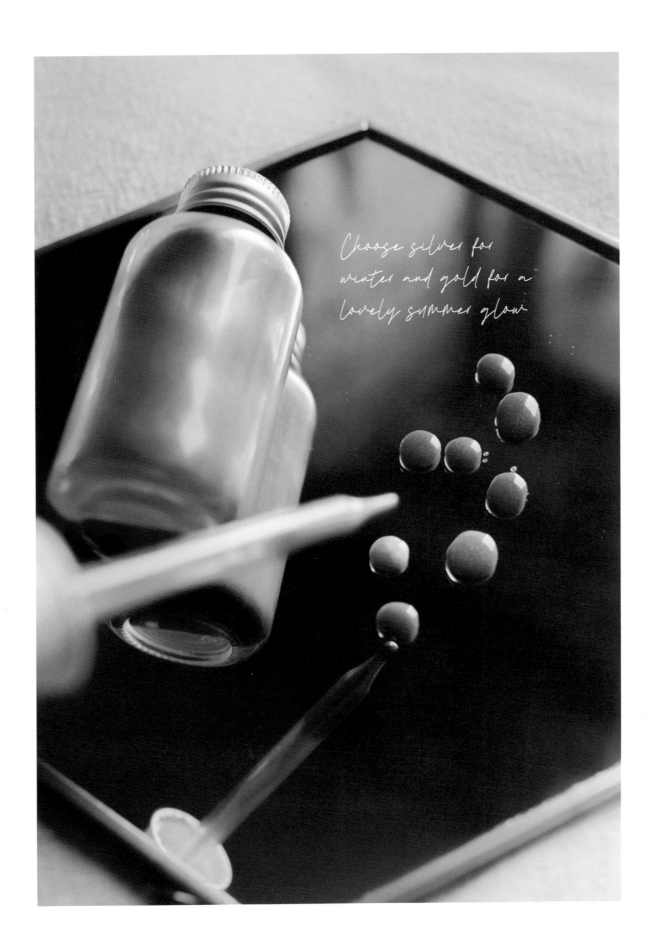

Choose silver for winter and gold for a lovely summer glow

liquid gold drops

These super simple liquid gold shimmer drops are perfect to add into your creams and moisturisers to give you a slight shimmer, or you can just pop it straight onto your cheekbones for a dewy golden glow.

What you'll need

■ ¼ tsp Vitamin E

■ 2 tbsp Sweet almond oil

■ 2 tsp Gold mica powder

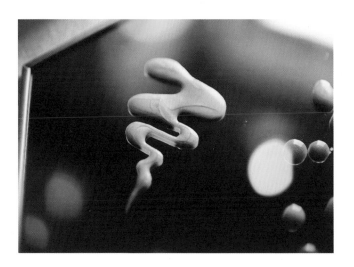

HOW TO MAKE

1. Pour the sweet almond oil and vitamin E into a small bowl.

2. Add the mica powder and stir with a spatula until completely combined.

3. Using a funnel, scoop every last drop of the mixture into a dropper bottle.

4. Your drops are now ready to use.

Emilie's tips

■ Try putting a drop on your finger and using it as a golden liquid eye shadow.

■ Remember to shake or stir your drops each time you use them to disperse the mica; it can tend to settle at the bottom of the container.

■ Pop a couple of drops into your palm while applying body butter for an all-over natural glow.

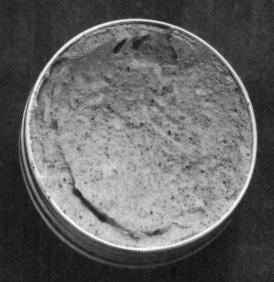
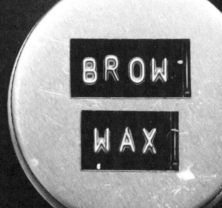

tinted eyebrow wax

I love to use a tinted wax as it shapes and colours your brows at the same time. This wax will last all day long, keeping your brows tinted, defined and tamed.

What you'll need

- 1 tsp Beeswax (use 3 tsp soya for a vegan alternative)
- 3 tsp Coconut oil
- ½ tsp Sweet almond oil
- ¼ tsp Cocoa powder
- ½ tsp Cinnamon powder
- Pinch Colour powder (see below)

HOW TO MAKE

1. Melt the wax and oil together in a bowl over a pan of boiling water.

2. Take it off the heat when completely melted and add in the sweet almond oil and your chosen colour of powder (your colour powder should be no more than 1 tsp once mixed).

3. Mix thoroughly until the colour is even.

4. Keep mixing until the mixture starts to become more solid and buttery before transferring into a tin.

HOW TO USE

Use an angled small brush, an old toothbrush or a clean old mascara wand to apply the wax.

When customising your wax colour, go a shade darker than you think. It will look dark in the tin, but much lighter when applied to your brows. You could also go colourless and just leave out the powders.

Emilie's tips

My colour suggestions

BLACK use ¾ tsp of activated charcoal and ¼ tsp of cocoa powder.

DARK BROWN use a mix of ½ tsp activated charcoal and ½ tsp cocoa powder.

MID BROWN use ¼ tsp cocoa powder and ¾ tsp cinnamon powder.

RED use 1 tsp cinnamon powder.

BLONDE use ¼ tsp turmeric powder with ¼ tsp cinnamon and ½ tsp ginger powder.

- Create your own blend by experimenting with a mixture of powders. Just make sure the powders combined create no more than 1 tsp of powder in total.

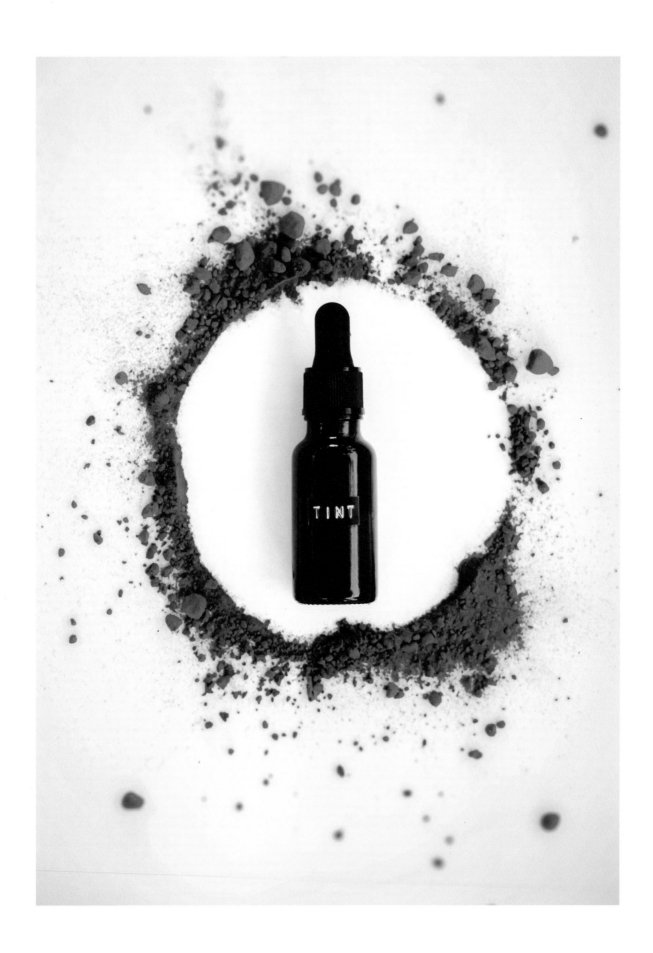

berry lip & cheek tint

If you've ever used a liquid lip and cheek stain then you'll know how long lasting and natural looking they are. I love them. You can customise your shade with this recipe, making the perfect colour for you. Once you've tried this tint you'll never reach for those expensive stains again!

What you'll need

- 1 tsp Aloe vera gel
- 1 tsp Glycerine
- 1 tsp Witch hazel
- ¼ tsp Beetroot powder
- ¼ tsp Cranberry powder

HOW TO MAKE

1. Combine the glycerine and aloe in a clean bowl.

2. Stir in the witch hazel.

3. Add in your chosen powder combination depending on your preferred colour choice.

4. Mix the powder until it is completely combined.

5. Spoon or pipette the mixture into a dropper bottle. It's then ready to use straight away.

Emilie's tips

- Beetroot creates more of a red tint and cranberry creates more of a deep pink tint so change the recipe to make the colour you want. You can also use dragon fruit powder for pink tints. My perfect combination is a half and half mixture that perfectly suits my skin tone.

- Beetroot contains powerful antioxidants to keep your skin looking young and supple.

- This recipe will last around two months, so make it in small batches.

- Use vegetable glycerine to make this recipe vegan and even more sustainable.

sustainable spa facial

There's nothing more luxurious than going for a facial, so I've created a sustainable facial spa session for you to make and enjoy yourself at home - all the luxury and none of the waste. You'll start with a steam session, followed by exfoliation and peel treatments, a relaxing face mask and finally a serum of your choice. You'll be amazed at how many of the ingredients in these recipes you have in your kitchen and garden.

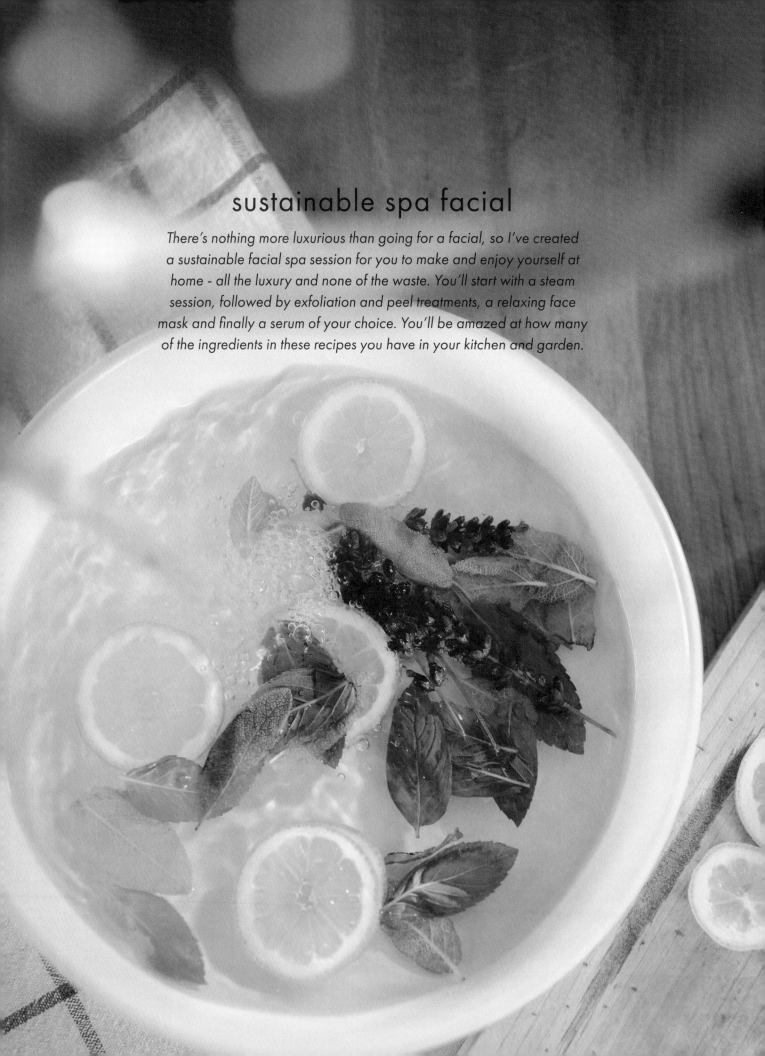

herbal facial steam

Steaming your skin is one of the best ways to clear blocked pores. The heat encourages your skin to sweat, helping to open your pores and get rid of the the dirt and grime that builds up on your skin. The fresh herbs and citrus ingredients smell fantastic and, more importantly, help to cleanse and brighten up your skin.

What you'll need

■ Freshly boiled water

■ 5 Lavender heads

■ Handful fresh sage & mint leaves

■ ½ Lemon thinly sliced

HOW TO MAKE

1. Pop a large bowl onto a steady surface.

2. Take your herbs and slap each of them in the palm of your hand. This helps to break down the plant cells and release their scents and oils.

3. Put all the herbs into a bowl with the sliced lemon and top it up with boiling water.

HOW TO USE

1. Position your face directly above the bowl and drape a towel over your head to create mini steam chamber.

2. Breathe the steam deeply through your nose for around 10 to 15 minutes.

3. When finished, rinse your skin with fresh warm water and pat dry.

Emilie's tips

■ If you've don't have herbs, swap for 1 drop of lavender and a drop of eucalyptus essential oil instead.

■ Dried herbs are a good alternative

■ Make sure to pop your spent herbs into the compost.

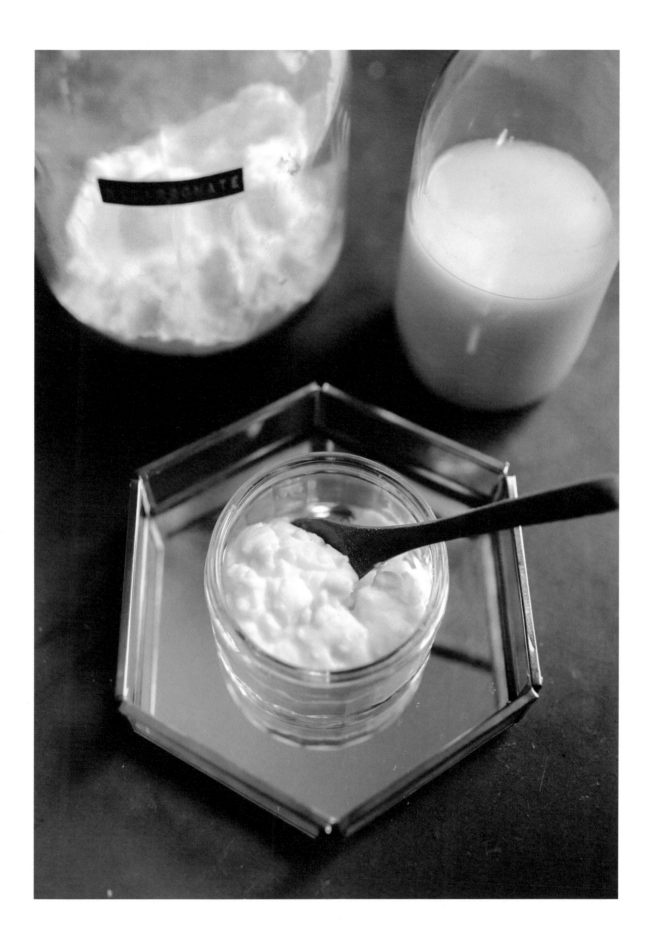

Step 2. Exfoliate

lactic acid dermabrasion

This treatment will remove dead skin cells and clear your pores of the grime that has been softened by the facial steaming, leaving your skin feeling silky. The fine bicarbonate powder will polish your skin, getting into every nook and cranny. The milk contains plenty of lactic acid, which is a great naturally acidic skin exfoliator to help increase cell renewal, reduce hyperpigmentation and smooth out fine lines.

What you'll need
- 4 tbsp Bicarbonate of soda
- 1 & ½ tbsp Milk

HOW TO MAKE

1. Measure our the bicarbonate of soda and milk into a bowl and mix together until smooth.

2. Use the mixture straight away.

HOW TO USE

1. Apply the dermabrasion cream onto your dry skin, working in circular motions over your face, taking care to avoid the eye area.

2. Keep working over problem areas like your t-zone for a few minutes.

2. Steam off with a hot muslin cloth or flannel and pat your face dry.

Emilie's tips

- For a vegan alternative, you can use oat milk which also contains lactic acid.

- For a stronger lactic acid content, use milk that is past its best as the acid will be more concentrated as the milk begins to ferment. Leave it as long as you dare!

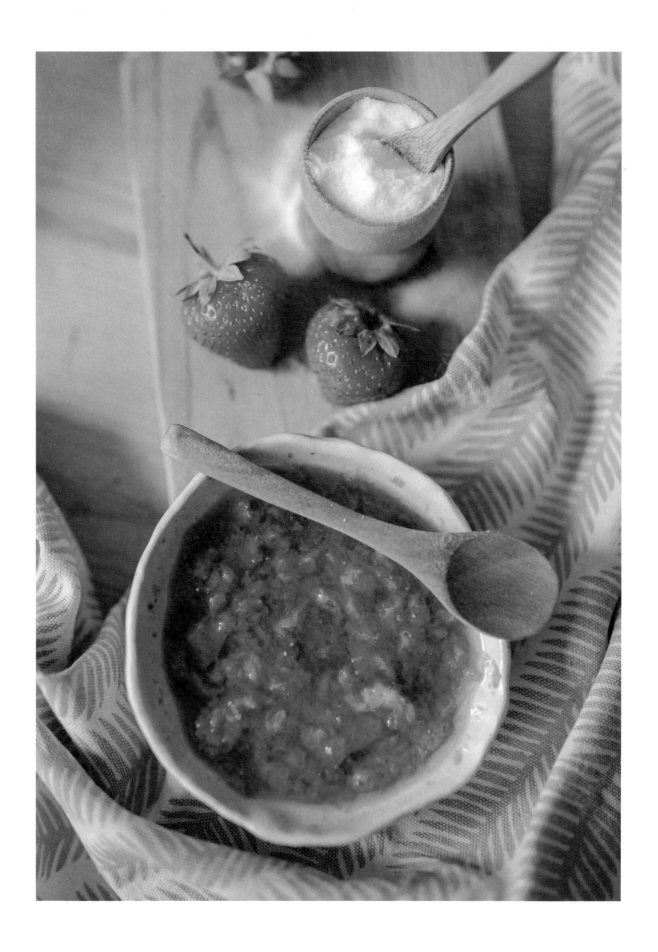

strawberries & sugar acid peel

Strawberries and sugar are normally reserved for my favourite dessert served with ice cream, but they also have a secret super power that is fantastic for your skin - glycolic acid. Derived from sugar cane, glycolic acid is used in luxury skin peels as it gently removes the top layer of dead skin cells, leaving you with lovely soft, fresh, glowing skin!

What you'll need

■ 4 or 5 Strawberries

■ 3 tsp Caster sugar

HOW TO MAKE

1. Blend the strawberries with a stick blender until liquid. Use a fork if you don't have a blender.

2. Add the caster sugar and mix until the ingredients are completely combined.

3. Pour the mixture into a small pan and pop it on a medium heat to melt the sugar.

4. Stir to keep the mixture moving around in the pan and don't let it come to the boil.

5. Once the sugar has dissolved, take the pan off the heat and leave it to cool down for a few minutes.

6. Once cool enough, it's ready to use. Strain out the strawberries if you prefer a smoother mixture.

HOW TO USE

Apply the peel to clean, dry skin, making sure you avoid the eye area. Let it work for 20 minutes before washing it off with warm water. You can use this mask once every 2 weeks; any more and it may irritate your skin.

Emilie's tips

■ Make sure to wear SPF for a day or so after using this peel as your skin may be more sensitive to the sun.

■ If strawberries are out of season swap out for other high acid fruits like apples in autumn and cranberries in the winter.

■ If you have strained your stawberries, these are fab on toast or swirled into yoghurt!

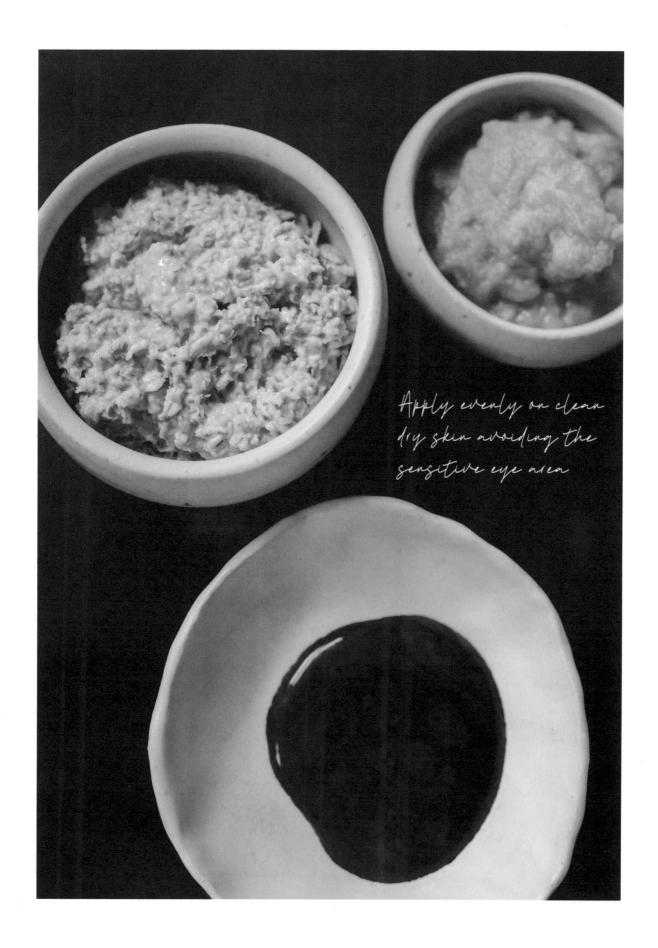

Apply evenly on clean
dry skin avoiding the
sensitive eye area

soothing oats & honey

Oats and honey are well known for their soothing effects on skin. Their calming qualities can help to soothe skin irritations and are perfect for using on dry, sensitive skin.

What you'll need
- ¼ cup Rolled oats
- 2 tbsp Runny honey

HOW TO MAKE

1. Whizz the oats in a blender or crush in a pestle and mortar until they are quite fine.

2. Slightly warm the honey in the microwave for 15 seconds before adding to the oat mixture.

3. Mix thoroughly to combine and apply straight away.

Emilie's tips
- Try and use local raw honey to be even more sustainable.
- Best for sensitive and dry skin.

anti-ageing carrot, honey & orange

This face mask is all about the carrot's antioxidant and vitamin properties, which brighten your skin, reducing fine lines and lightening age spots. Carrots contain Vitamin A which stimulates the production of collagen which helps with anti-ageing.

What you'll need
- 1 Carrot - medium sized
- 1 Orange - small, grated peel
- 1 tbsp Honey

HOW TO MAKE

1. Wash and thinly slice the carrot, before steaming it until it is cooked through.
2. Once the carrot is cooked, mash it into a paste.
3. Add in the grated orange and honey, mixing well.
4. Once combined, it's ready to use!

Emilie's tips
- The vitamin C in carrots & oranges help brighten your skin.
- This is best for mature, oily or sun-damaged skin.

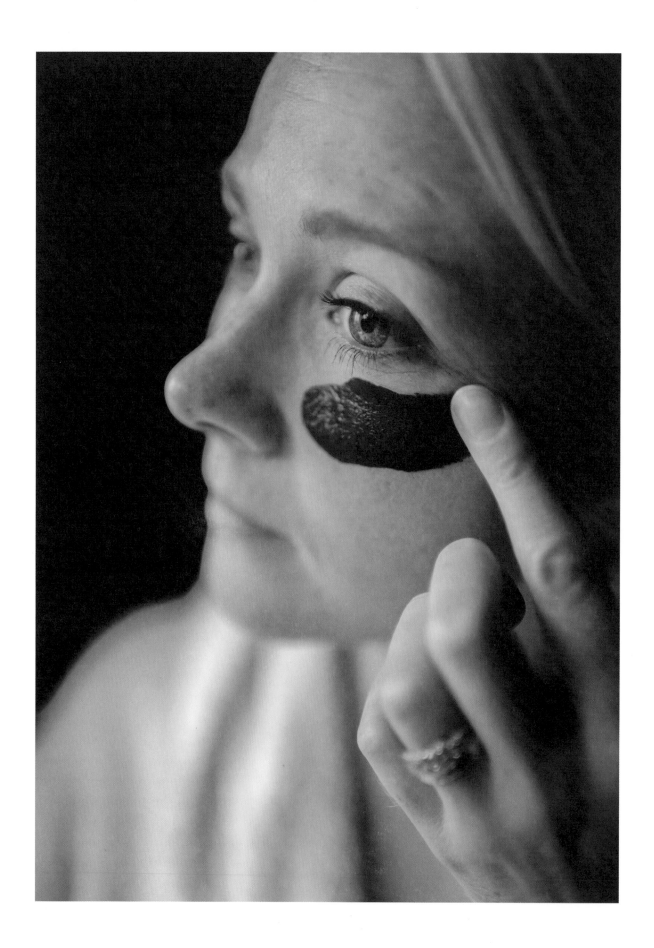

detoxing charcoal & clay

This detoxifying face mask uses activated charcoal and clay to draw out impurities and toxins; great for removing blackheads and tightening your pores. It's the perfect mask if you suffer from oily skin, clogged pores or regular breakouts. The tea tree oil in this recipe is antibacterial and helps prevent bacteria from settling on your skin, which can lead to breakouts.

What you'll need

■ 2 tsp Kaolin clay

■ ¼ tsp Activated charcoal

■ ½ tsp Distilled water

■ 5 drops Sweet almond oil

■ 3 drops Tea tree essential oil

HOW TO MAKE

1. Measure the charcoal and clay into a small bowl.

2. Add the water and oil and mix until smooth.

3. Drop in your tea tree oil and mix again.

4. You're ready to use.

Emilie's tips

■ This mask is best for oily and combination skin that is prone to breakouts.

■ This mask works best when slightly damp, so to keep it working on your skin, try spritzing your face with water to stop it drying out.

Step 5. Moisturising face serum

This last step is to moisturise your now fully pampered skin. Try making my favourite anti-ageing face serum on Page 40, or just use sweet almond oil mixed with a few drops of lavender and frankincense essential oil to make a simple moisturiser which will leave your skin feeling pampered, moisturised and smelling gorgeous.

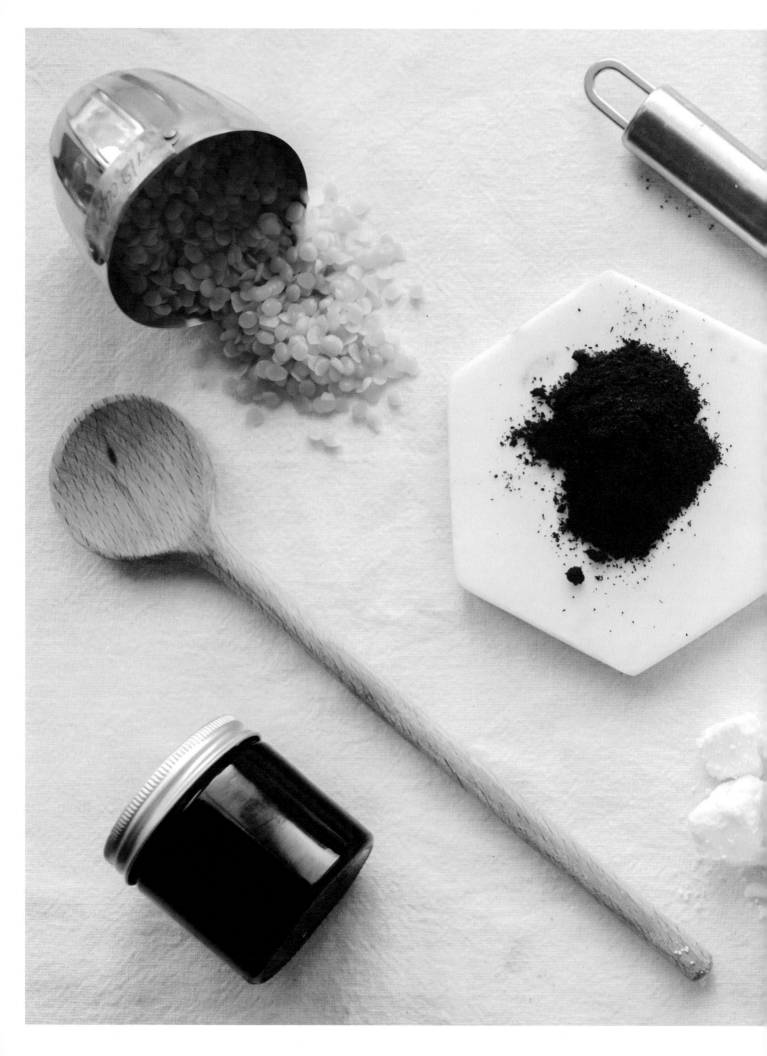

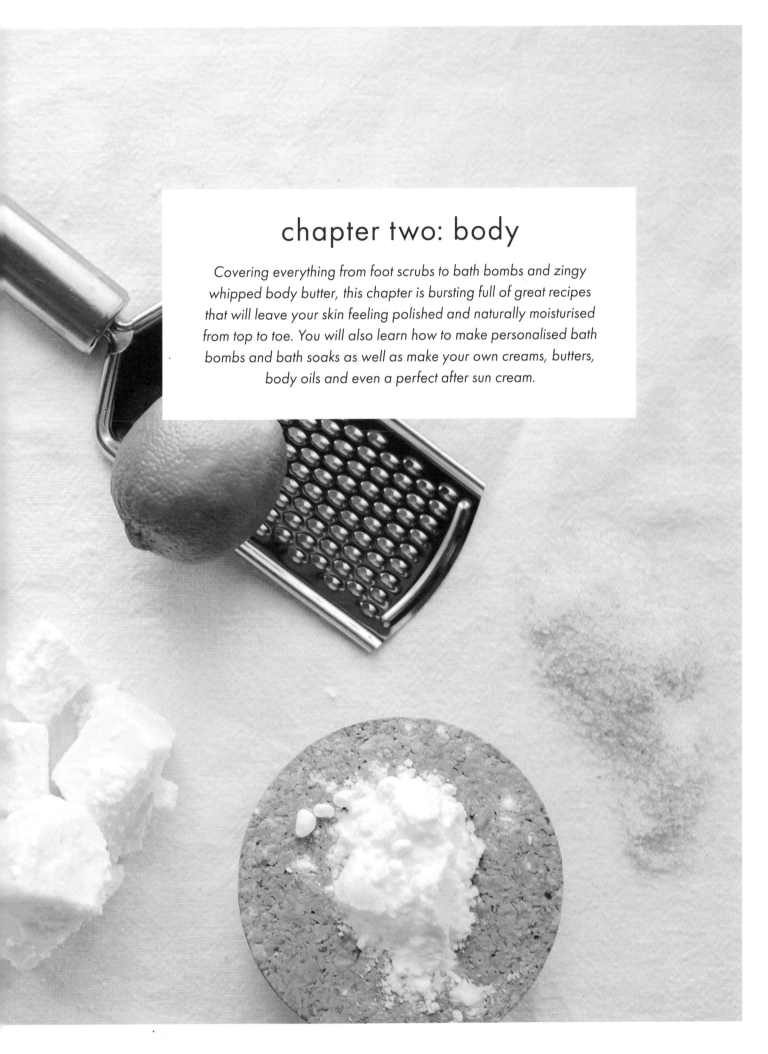

chapter two: body

Covering everything from foot scrubs to bath bombs and zingy whipped body butter, this chapter is bursting full of great recipes that will leave your skin feeling polished and naturally moisturised from top to toe. You will also learn how to make personalised bath bombs and bath soaks as well as make your own creams, butters, body oils and even a perfect after sun cream.

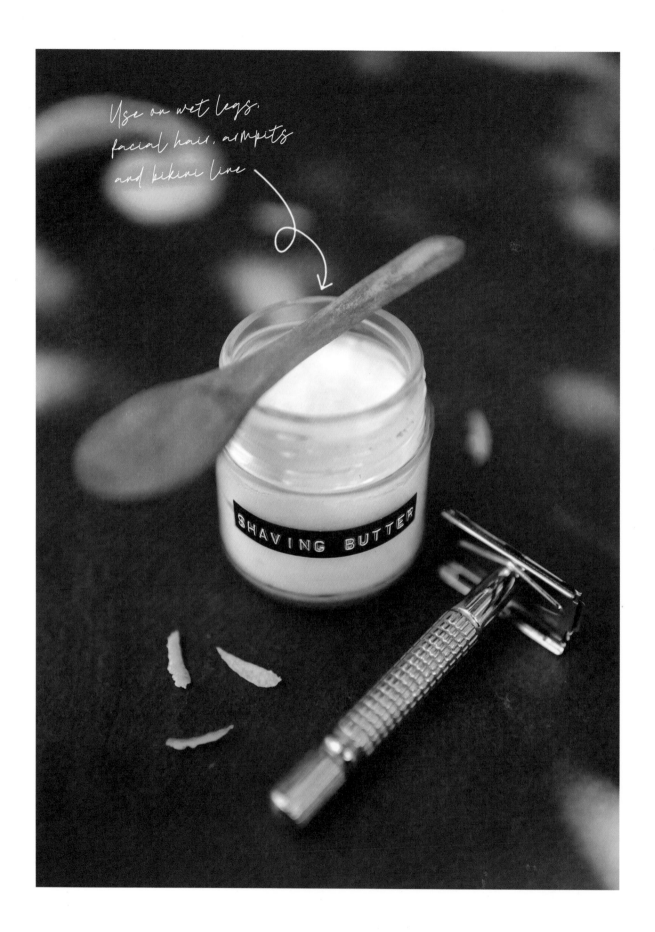

Use on wet legs, facial hair, armpits and bikini line

orange & ginger shaving butter

After making the switch to a reusable safety razor (it's the best shave you'll ever have; you should definitely try them) I knew I had to go zero waste with my shaving butter too. This shaving butter is creamy, rich and fluffy and leaves your skin supple and velvety after a lovely close shave.

What you'll need

- ¼ cup Sweet almond oil
- ¼ cup Coconut oil
- ¼ cup Cocoa butter
- 3 tbsp Castile soap
- 10 drops Orange essential oil
- 5 drops Ginger essential oil

HOW TO MAKE

1. Place a bowl over a pan of water and add in all of the oils and butters. Mix them up until they are completely melted.

2. Take the bowl off the heat and set the mixture to one side to cool for 15 minutes or so. You can speed this process up by popping the mixture in the fridge for 5 minutes until it starts to look opaque and begins to set.

3. Using a whisk (electric if you have one) whip the mixture and then add in the castile soap and essential oils.

4. Whip the mixture again until the soap and oils are completely blended and the mixture is light and fluffy. This may take a while if you are using a hand whisk. Try and get as much air as possible into the mixture when whipping.

5. Transfer your mixture into a clean sterilised jar and it's ready to be used!

Emilie's tips

- Use a small spoon to apply the butter to your skin. This helps to avoid getting water into the mixture which could cause it to go mouldy.
- Massage a small amount of the butter into your skin until it begins to go milky. You can then start to shave, rinsing the razor often. When finished rinse and pat your skin dry. There is no need to apply a moisturiser; your skin will be feeling super moisturised and silky smooth.
- Disposable razors are non-recyclable. By switching to a safety razor, you never have to buy a disposable single-use plastic razor again.

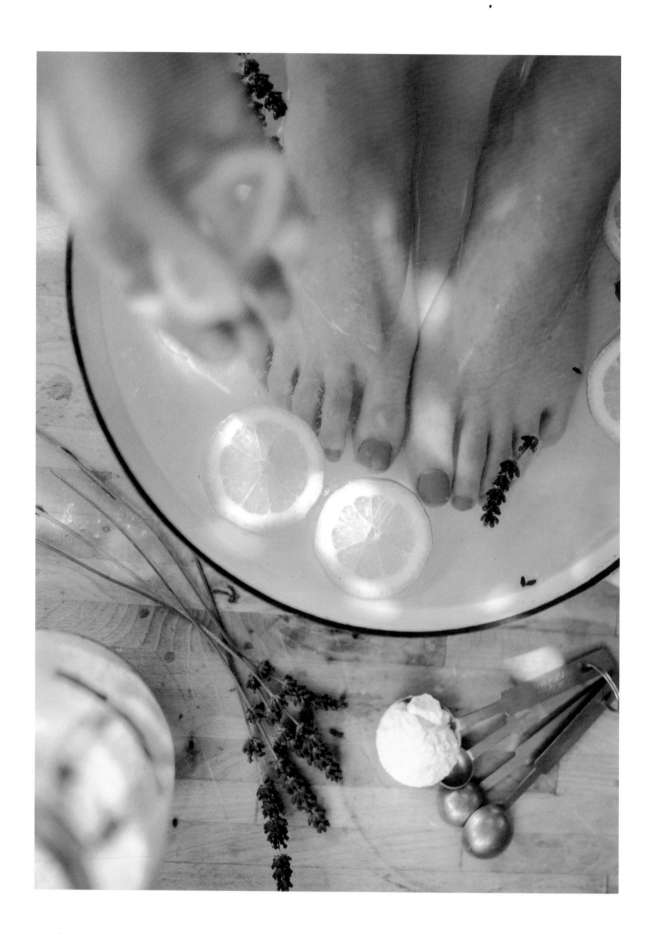

fizzy lavender & lemon foot soak

It's always best to give your feet a good soak and soften up any dry skin before applying a scrub to get the best effect. This skin softening foot soak smells heavenly - so take some time for yourself, breathe deeply and soak your tootsies!

What you'll need

- ■ 4 tbsp Bicarbonate of soda
- ■ 1 Lemon, sliced
- ■ 5 cups Warm water
- ■ 3 drops Lavender essential oil

HOW TO MAKE

1. Grab a large container. Something like an old casserole dish will do the job.

2. Measure out the bicarbonate of soda and top up with warm water.

3. Slice the lemon into 1cm rounds and squeeze lightly before dropping into the water. Watch them fizz!

4. Add the lavender essential oil and swish the water around to disperse it evenly.

5. Grab a book or pop your favourite podcast on, sink your feet into your soak and relax for 20 minutes.

Emilie's tips

- ■ Bicarbonate of soda and lemon make the fizz in this recipe and when combined make a great anti fungal soak.
- ■ Squeeze the lemon rounds with your toes for extra fizzy bursts as they soak.
- ■ Follow this soak with my peppermint & lime foot scrub and body butter for the loveliest softest feet.

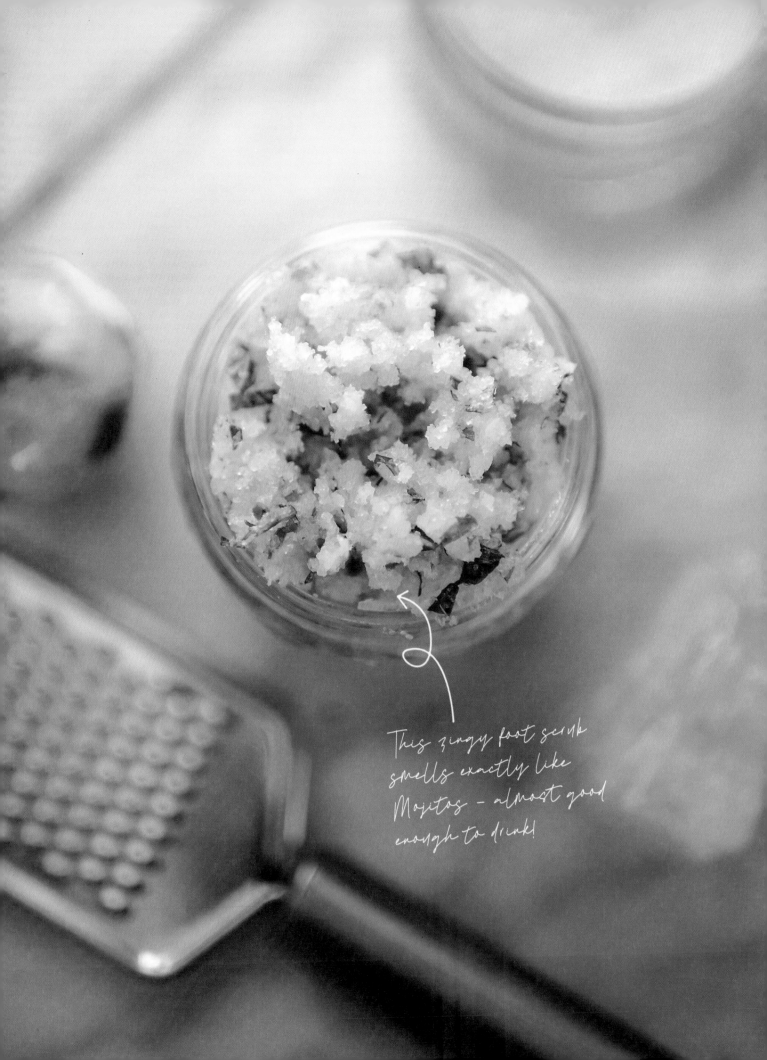

This zingy foot scrub smells exactly like Mojitos – almost good enough to drink!

peppermint & lime foot salt scrub

After making this fresh, zingy foot scrub you'll never reach for a pre-made one again. The fresh mint not only creates an odour-eliminating scent, but actually helps to reduce sweating! The salt is the exfoliator in this recipe and also helps to improve circulation.

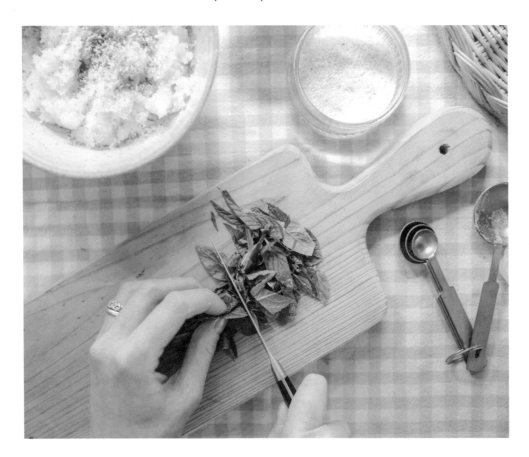

What you'll need

- ½ cup Coconut oil

- 3 tbsp pink Himalayan salt

- 1 cup Granulated sugar

- 4 sprigs Fresh mint, chopped

- 1 Lime, grated

Emilie's tip

- To make this recipe shelf stable you can swap the fresh ingredients for essential oils. Simply add in drops of lime essential oil and 8 drops of peppermint.

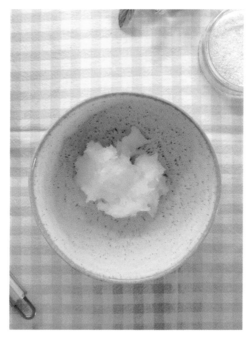

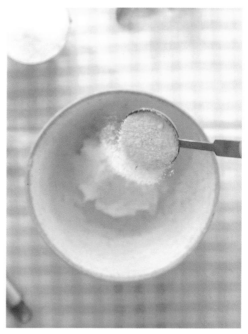

1. Scoop the coconut oil into a bowl and leave for a few minutes to soften slightly.

2. Add in the pink Himalayan salt, which is packed full of minerals, great for your skin.

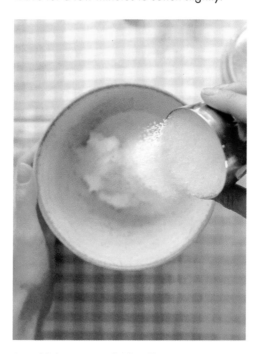

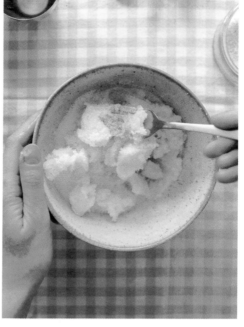

3. Add the sugar which will attract moisture from the air to keep your feet feeling supple.

4. Combine the ingredients by mashing with a fork. Don't worry if it's lumpy at this stage.

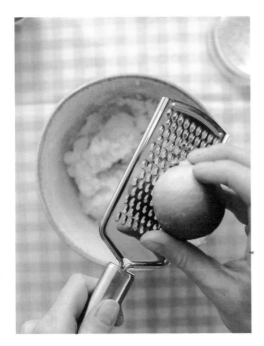

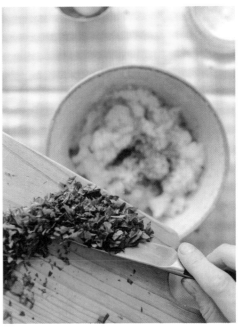

5. Add the lime zest and juice. Don't forget to compost the lime and pips.

6. Chop the mint and add to the mixture to give your scrub a fresh uplifting scent.

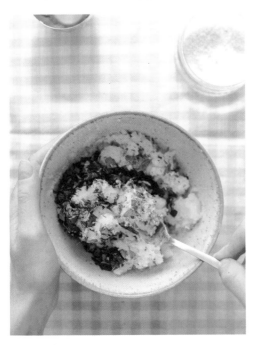

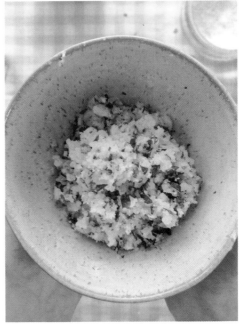

7. Mix everything together, using a fork to squish any big lumps of coconut oil.

8. Transfer your mixture into a clean glass jar and use within a week.

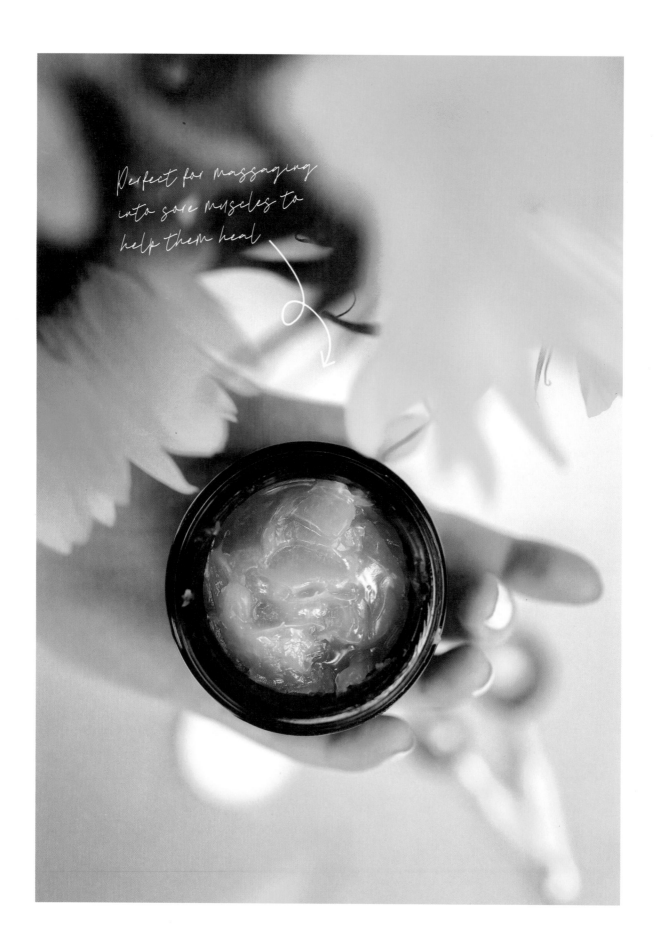

Perfect for massaging
into sore muscles to
help them heal

spicy muscle rub

This rub includes a mixture of essential oils which all play a vital part in making this rub really work on soothing your muscles. Perfect for after a gym work out or to relax after a long day at work.

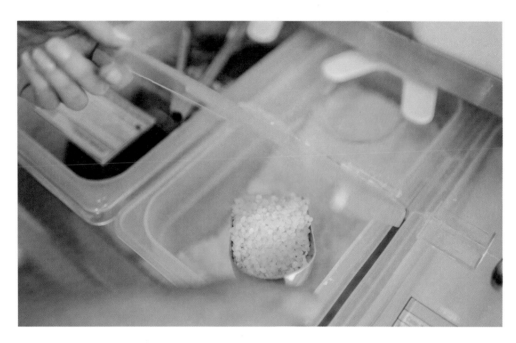

What you'll need

- ⅓ cup Olive Oil

- ½ cup Shea butter

- 2 tbsp Beeswax pellets

- Essential oils
  20 drops of camphor
  20 drops of peppermint
  10 drops of eucalyptus
  10 drops of cinnamon
  10 drops of clove

Camphor Used to help increase the blood flow where it is applied helping to reduce inflammation, swelling and pain.
Peppermint Causes the skin to fluctuate between feeling cool and hot which helps to distract you from immediate pain. It also brings blood to the surface, speeding up the healing process.
Cinnamon & Eucalyptus Both are anti-inflammatory and can help reduce swelling and soothe sore muscles.
Clove Has a numbing effect which can help soothe pain almost immediately.

Emilie's tip

- Apply a pea-sized amount to the area of pain and massage it in. I love to massage this into my neck and shoulders after a day of desk-work and into my knees before a long run.

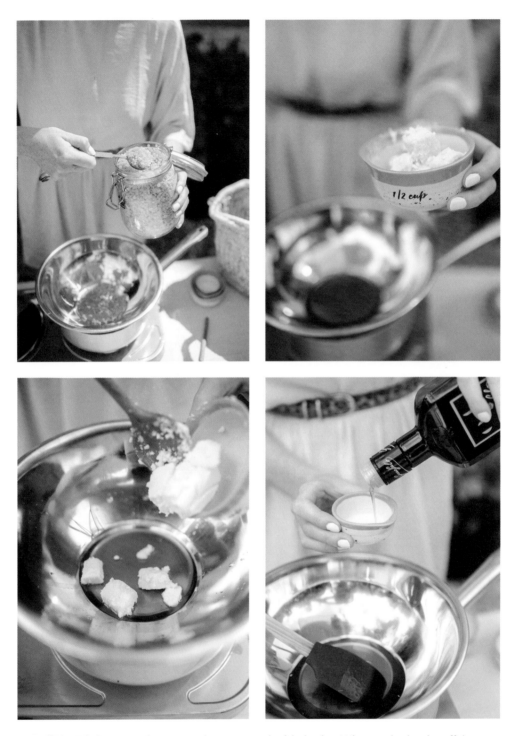

1. Melt the oil, butter and wax together using a double boiler. When melted, take off the heat and allow the mixture to cool for a few minutes.

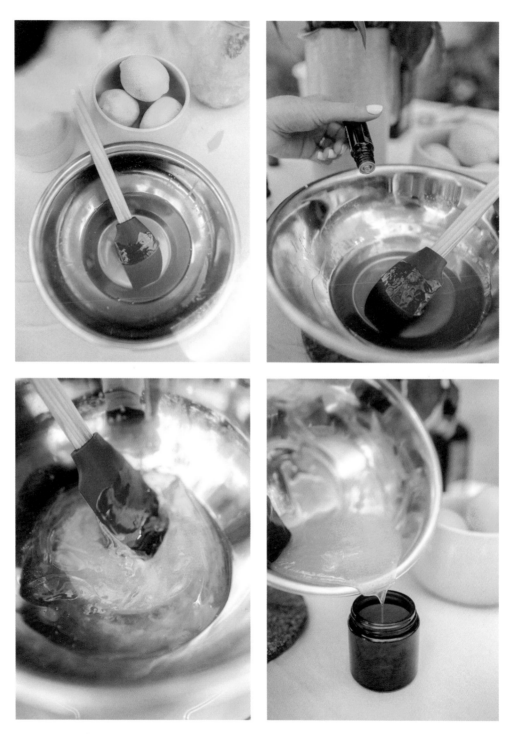

2. Add all of the essential oils and stir to combine. **3.** Pour the mixture into your chosen container and leave to set overnight or pop in the fridge for an hour or so.

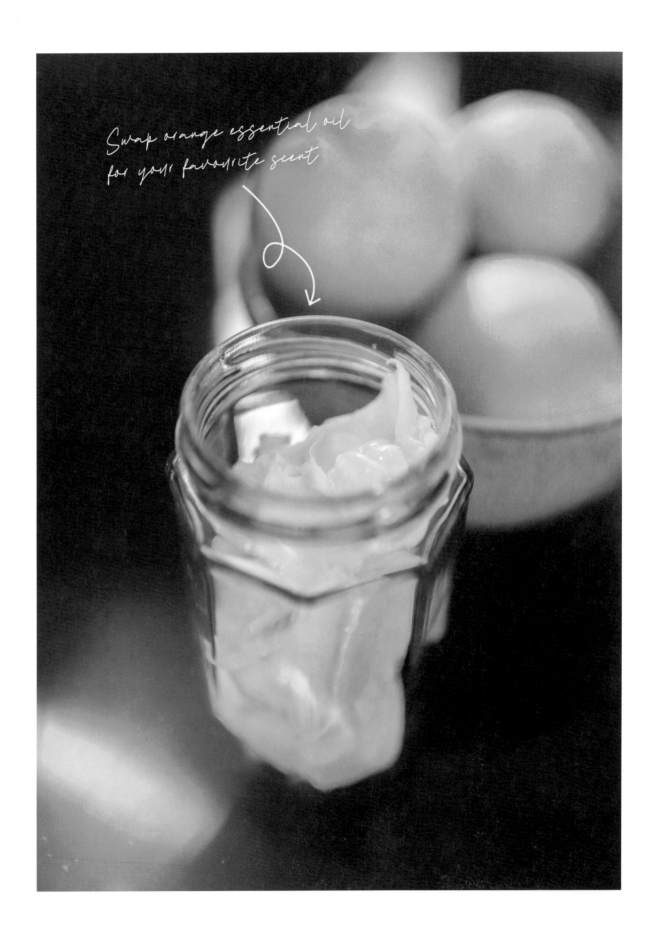

Swap orange essential oil for your favourite scent

whipped sweet orange body butter

This is a rich, whipped moisturiser and works best on dry skin. It is great for use all over your body; I love to use it on my legs, hands and elbows. The orange essential oil scent is zingy and uplifting, making this the perfect post shower, morning body butter.

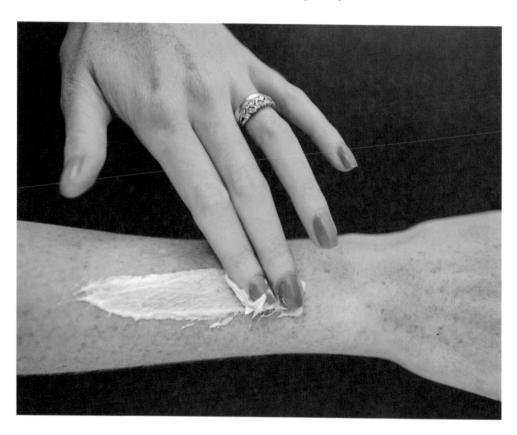

What you'll need

- 3 tbsp Sweet almond oil

- 2 tbsp Coconut oil

- 2 tbsp Beeswax

- 1 tbsp Shea butter

- 10 drops Orange essential oil

HOW TO USE

You can also use this body butter as a face night cream but only use a small amount as it is very rich; a little goes a long way. This body butter will last around 6 months if kept in a cool dark place.

Emilie's tip

- Perfect for using on dry skin, I love to slather my legs in this during the winter months to keep them moisturised and soft.

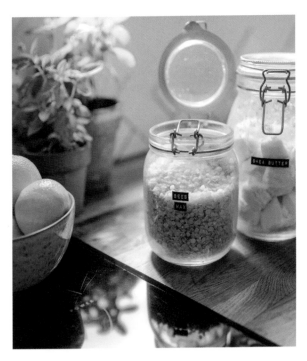

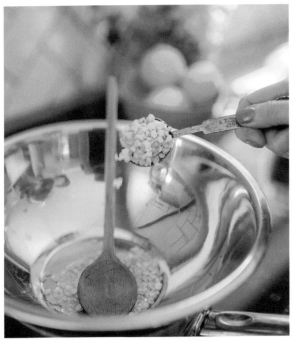

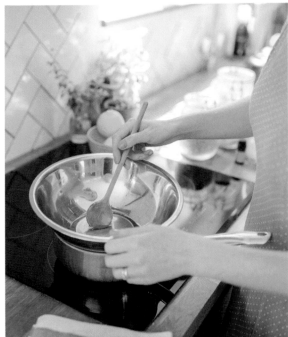

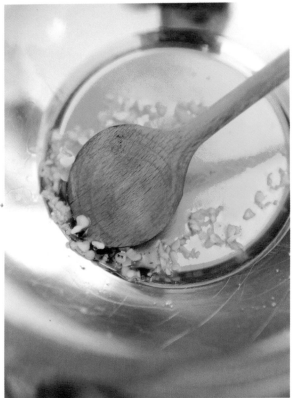

1. Melt the beeswax, coconut oil and shea butter in a non-plastic bowl over a pan of water or alternatively warm in the microwave in 30 second bursts.

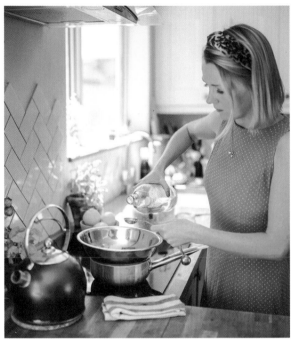

2. Leave to cool slightly and add in the sweet almond oil, mixing it in quickly and thoroughly to combine.

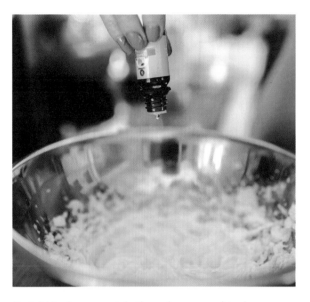

3. Add in the essential oils and start to whip the mixture. You can use a hand whisk or an electric whisk. An electric whisk will be quicker. Regularly scrape the mixture down from the sides to prevent any lumps from forming.

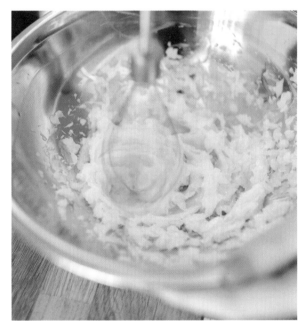

4. Keep whisking continuously until the mixture turns opaque and then light and fluffy.

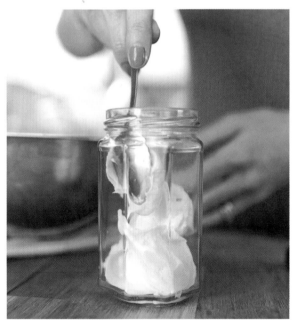

5. Once creamy and almost set, transfer the moisturiser into a sealed sterilised container.

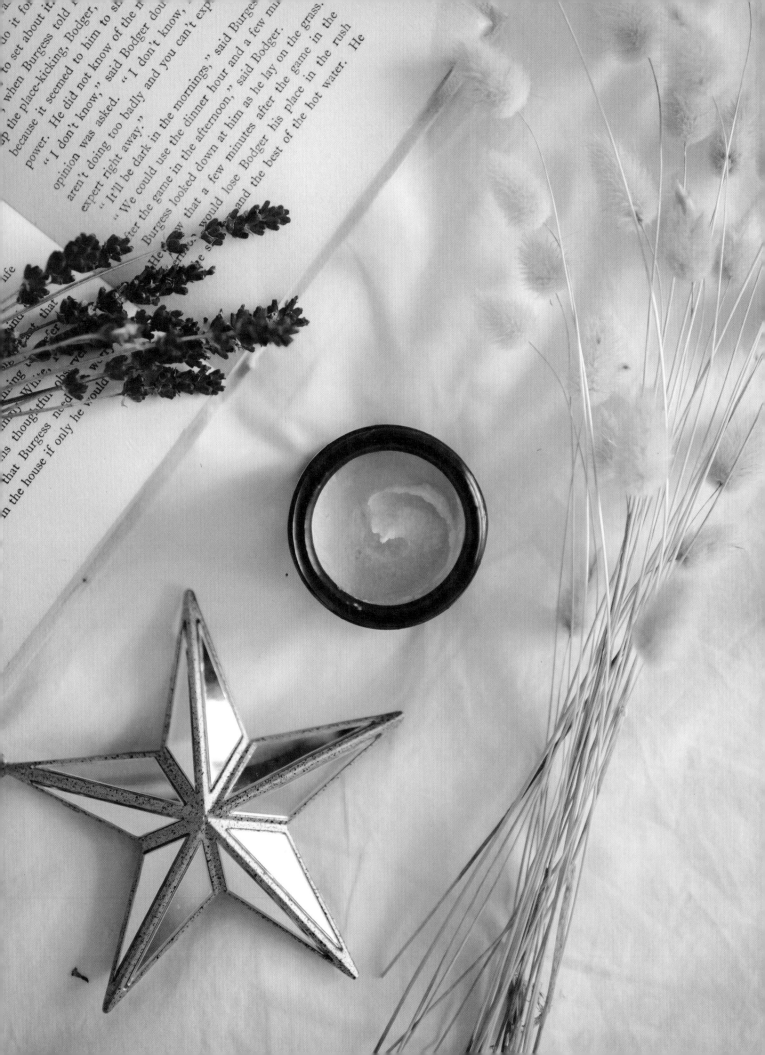

up it for
to set about it.
when Burgess told
the place-kicking, Bodger,
because it seemed to him to st.
power. He did not know of the n
"I don't know," said Bodger dou
opinion was asked. "I don't know,
aren't doing too badly and you can't exp
expert right away."
"It'll be dark in the mornings," said Burgess
"We could use the game in the dinner hour and a few mi
after the game in the afternoon," said Bodger.
Burgess looked down at him as he lay on the grass.
that a few minutes after the game in the rush
would lose Bodger his place in the
and the best of the hot water. He

lavender night time hand salve

The beeswax in this hand salve is naturally antibacterial, as is the coconut oil. The naturally calming and antibacterial lavender essential oil in this recipe makes it a great natural healing salve for any cuts or grazes. The lovely scent makes it a relaxing night time hand salve. I love to slather it all over my hands and breathe it in before dropping off to sleep – it's so relaxing.

What you'll need

■ 2 tbsp Shea butter

■ 1 ½ tsp Beeswax

■ 1 tbsp Sweet almond oil

■ 8 drops Lavender essential oil

HOW TO MAKE

1. Melt the wax and shea butter in a non-plastic bowl over a pan of water.

2. Add in the sweet almond oil and mix it up to combine.

3. Take off the heat and leave to cool for 2 minutes before adding in the essential oils. Stir to distribute them evenly.

4. Carefully pour the liquid salve into a sealed sterilised container and leave to set overnight. To speed this process up you can pop it into the fridge for an hour with the lid off.

Emilie's tips

■ This is a rich moisturising salve and works best when used on dry skin. It is great for dry hands, knees, elbows, feet or anywhere that needs some extra TLC. It is a staple for the winter months when our skin is dried out from the cold weather and central heating.

■ I like to massage this salve into my hands and feet in the evening before bed and then leave them to soak up all that goodness overnight.

■ This mixture will last 12 months if kept in a cool dark place.

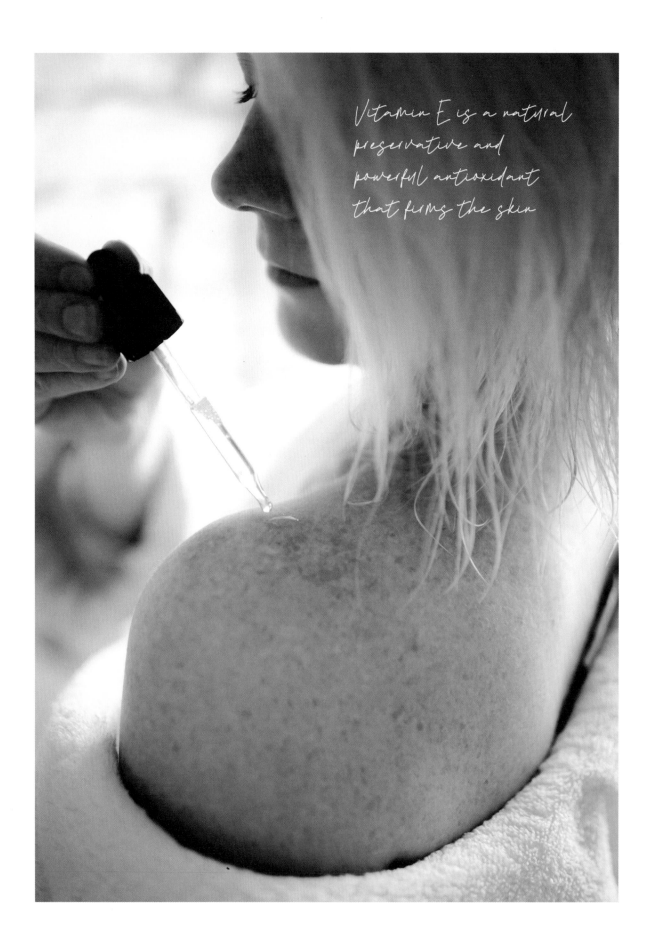

Vitamin E is a natural preservative and powerful antioxidant that firms the skin

toning body oil

I love to use a light body oil as an all-over moisturiser after my morning shower. This recipe is so easy and quickly absorbed into your skin. All the organic ingredients can easily be sourced as Soil Association approved. This is the perfect, affordable, simple, sustainable body oil.

What you'll need

- 1 cup Sweet almond oil
- 2 tbsp Vitamin E oil
- 20 drops Rosemary essential oil
- 10 drops Frankincense essential oil
- 5 drops Clove essential oil

HOW TO MAKE

1. Find your favourite container. Try to use a tinted glass container to help preserve the essential oils structure.

2. Put all of the ingredients straight into the container and shake well to combine them.

3. That's it! Ready to go!

Emilie's tips

- Rosemary helps to increase blood circulation, fights cellulite and brightens the skin.
- Frankincense has many amazing benefits for your skin including improving elasticity.
- Clove helps to firm and tighten the skin, remove dead skin cells and reduce the appearance of fine lines and wrinkles!

Take time to pamper
your nails with this
lovely nourishing oil

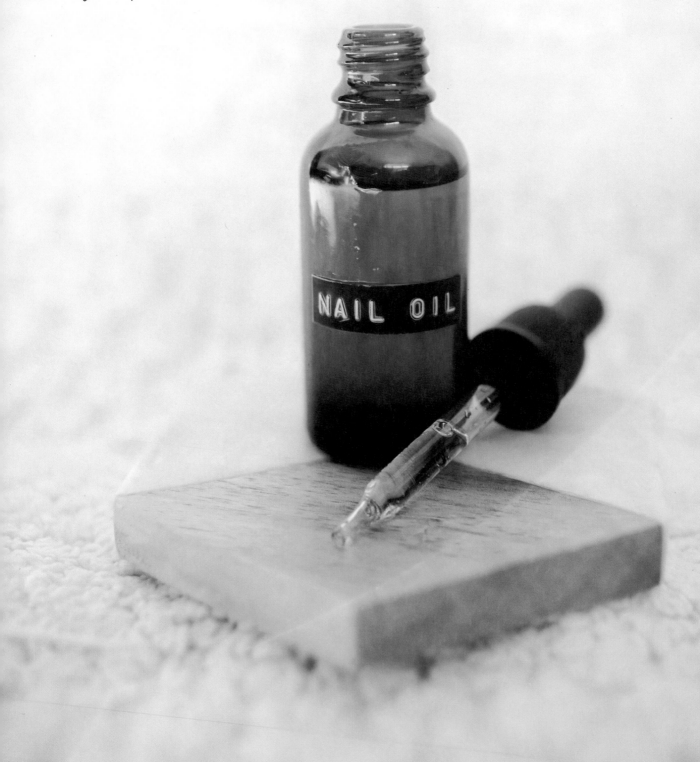

nail oil

This nail oil recipe is so quick and easy to make. It only uses three ingredients, which all help to nourish you nails as well as lift any stains from gardening or wearing dark nail polish.

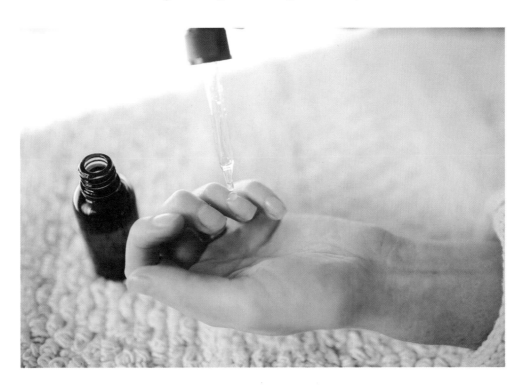

What you'll need

■ 3 tsp Jojoba oil

■ 1 tsp Sweet almond oil

■ 5 drops Lavender essential oil

■ 5 drops Lemon essential oil

HOW TO MAKE

1. Pour the oils into the container.

2. Add in the essential oils and shake to mix together.

3. You're ready to use!

Emilie's tips

■ The lavender is antibacterial and can help naturally heal any damage to your nails and the skin around it. The lemon essential oil will help to lift any stains on your nail surface.

■ I like to store my nail oil in a dropper bottle so I can use just the right amount. Dab the oil on your nail and cuticle bed and rub the oil into your nails and hands.

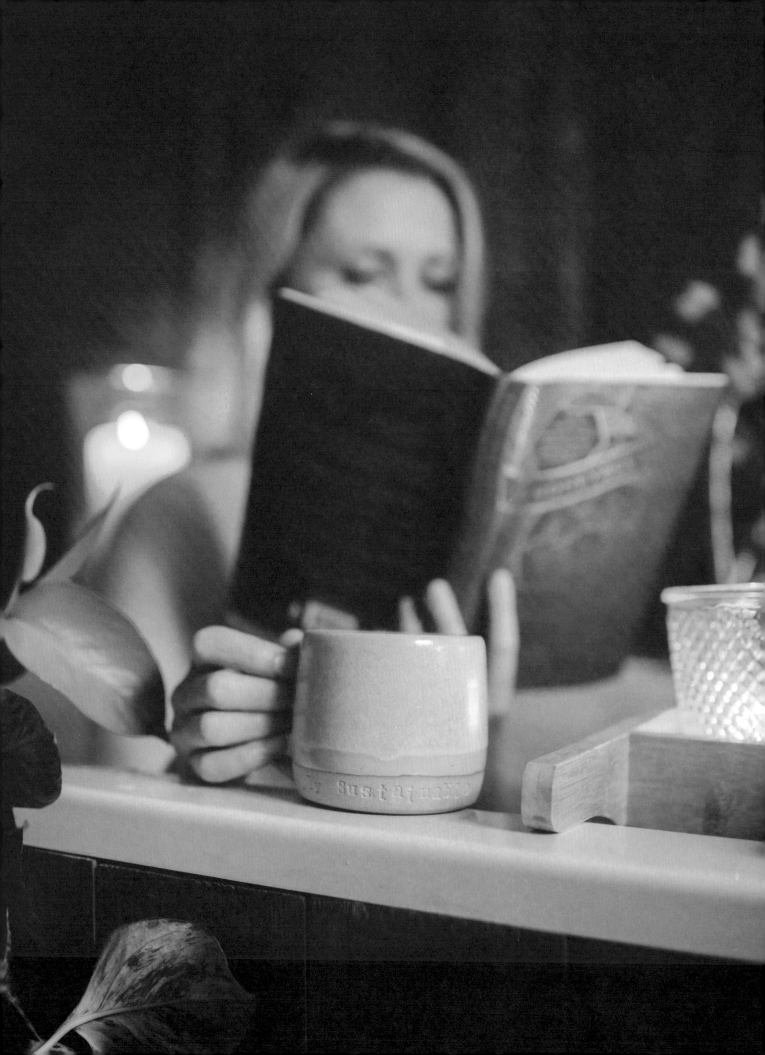

bath soaks

Bath soaks are one of the oldest forms of skin care. It's even said that Cleopatra used to bathe in milk and honey to keep her skin nourished thousands of years ago. These soaks are simple to make, leaving you plenty of time to relax in a hot scented bath.

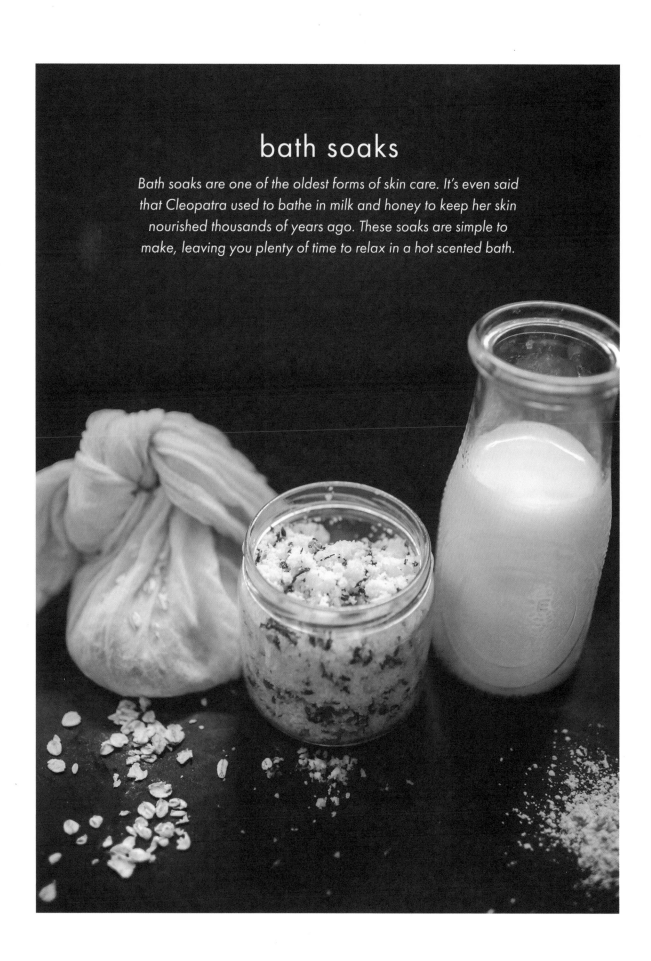

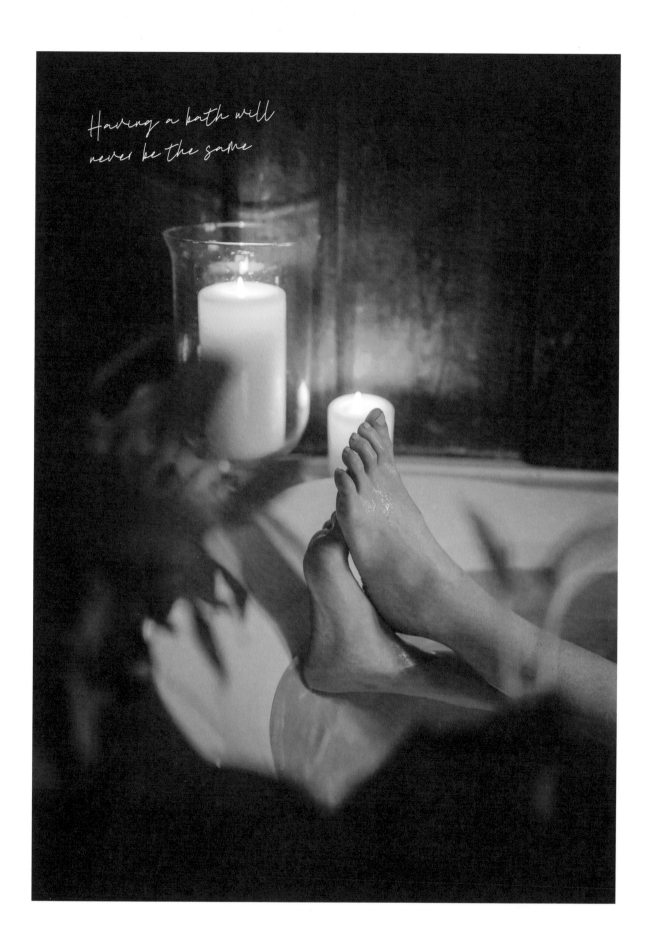

Having a bath will
never be the same

Egyptian milk & honey bath soak

Based on Cleopatra's favourite bath time recipe, this soak will help you wind down after a long day. All these bath soaks have different properties and help nourish your skin and body in different ways. Some need to be used straight away and some can be stored in a glass jar for months.

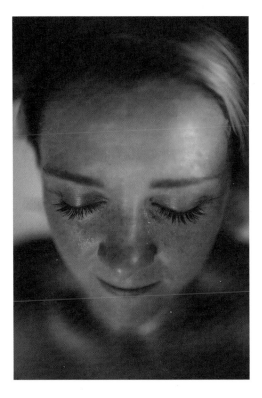 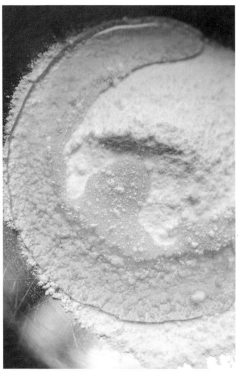

What you'll need

- ½ cup Milk powder
- 3 tbsp Honey
- 2 drops Lavender essential oil

Bath soaks make great gifts. Get experimental and switch up some of the scents to create your own personal blend. The lactic acid in milk helps to cleanse and remove dead skin cells, leaving your skin silky smooth and making you feeling as radiant as Cleopatra herself.

You can swap the powdered milk for fresh milk or switch to oat milk and agave syrup for a vegan alternative.

Pour your ingredients directly into your bath and stir to combine. Use immediately.

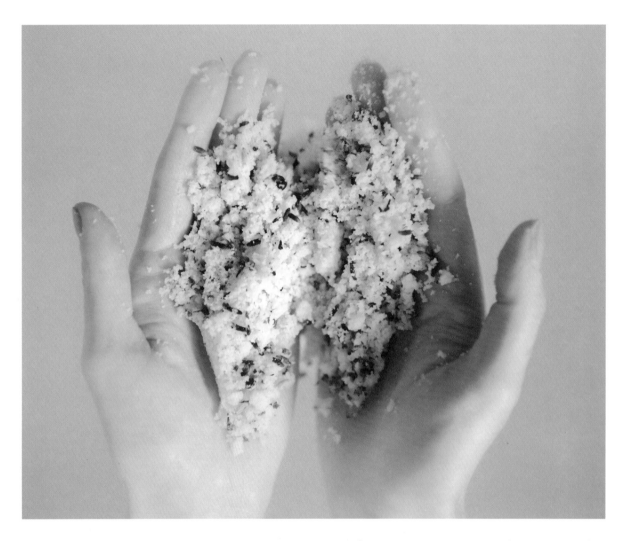

relaxing lavender & eucalyptus muscle soak

What you'll need

- ½ cup Epsom salts

- ¼ cup Bicarbonate of soda

- 2 tbsp Pink Himalayan salt

- 1 tbsp Jojoba oil

- 3 drops Lavender essential oil

- 2 drops Eucalyptus essential oil

The Epsom salts help to relax your muscles while the bicarbonate of soda and salt soften and rejuvenate your skin. Remember to breathe deeply while you're in the bath. The essential oils in the soak will make you feel as if you are in a spa and have great relaxation properties that are enhanced by controlled, deep breathing.

Store this recipe in a clean glass jar for up to a year.

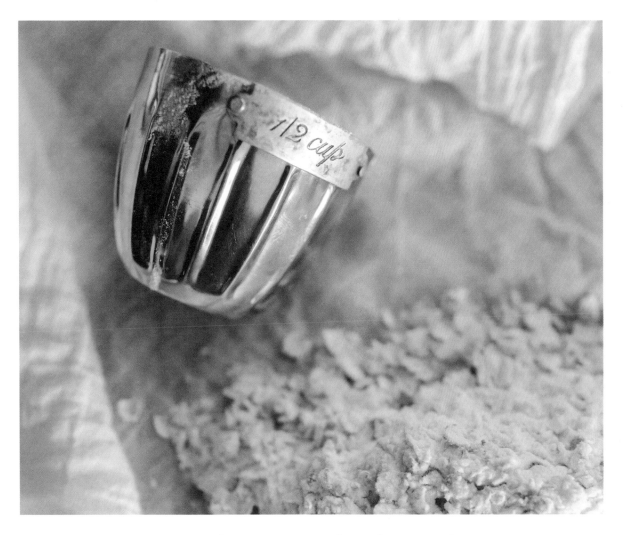

soothing oat bath soak

What you'll need

- ½ cup Rolled oats
- ¼ cup Bicarbonate of soda
- 5 drops Ylang ylang essential oil

Oats are fantastic for moisturising and soothing, while the bicarbonate of soda softens and neutralises the pH of your skin, which helps to soothe irritations. Ylang ylang has a beautiful floral scent and works wonders on improving your skins elasticity and tone.

Store this recipe in a clean glass jar for up to 6 months.

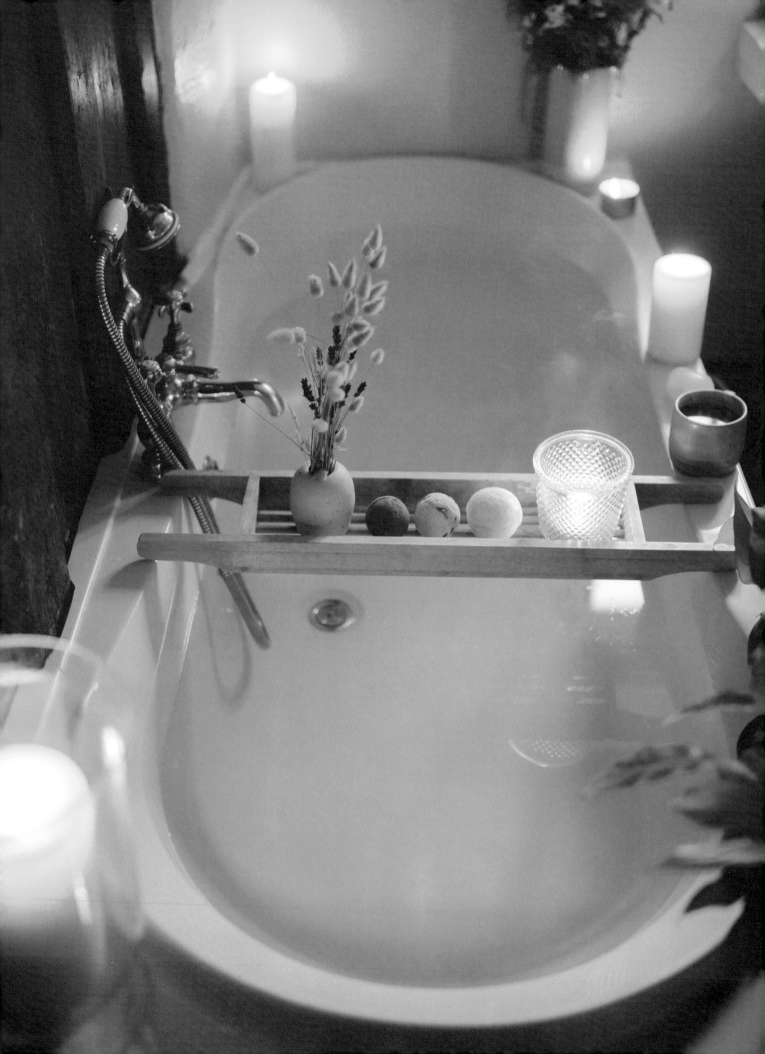

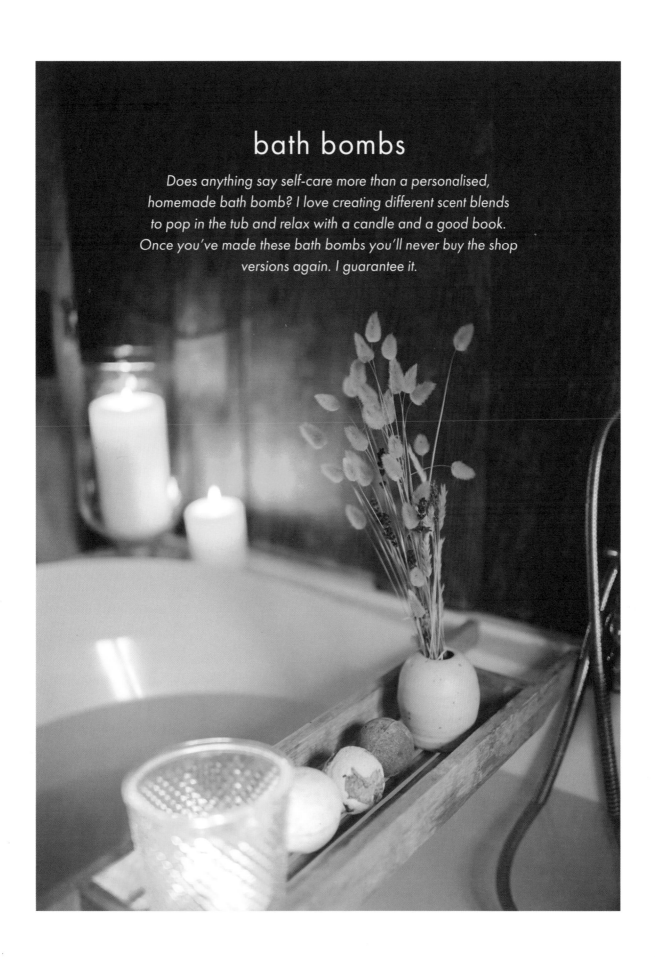

bath bombs

Does anything say self-care more than a personalised, homemade bath bomb? I love creating different scent blends to pop in the tub and relax with a candle and a good book. Once you've made these bath bombs you'll never buy the shop versions again. I guarantee it.

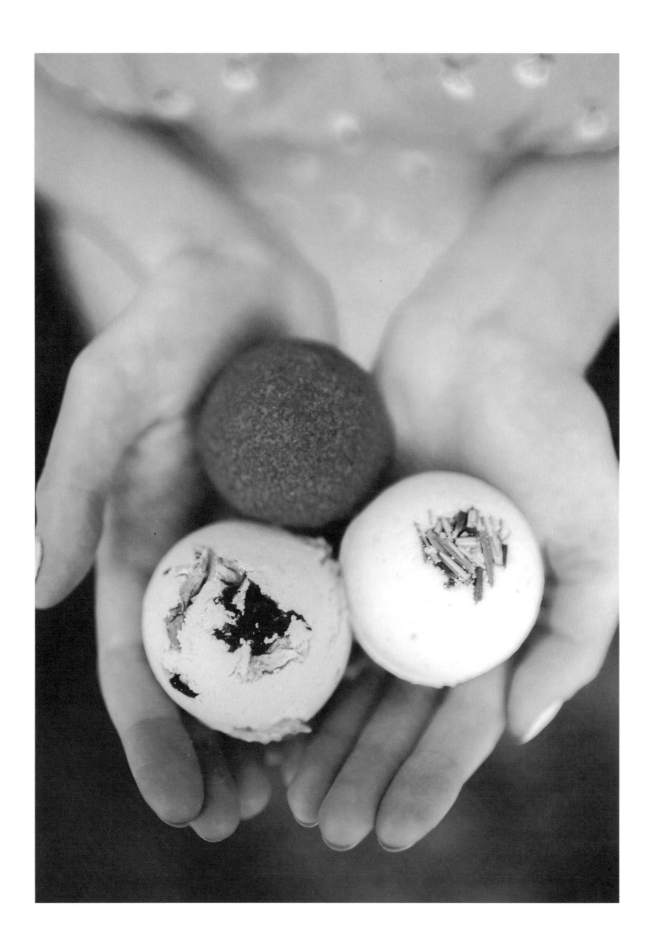

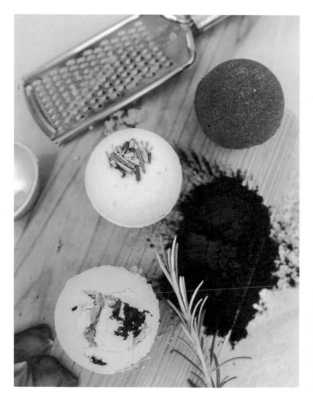

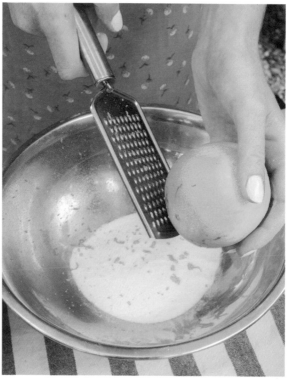

What you'll need

- 1 cup Bicarbonate of soda
- ⅓ cup Citric acid
- 1 tbsp Pink French clay (optional to add colour)
- 1 ½ tbsp Rose petals - dried
- ½ tsp Cocoa butter
- 7 drops Rose geranium essential oil
- ½ tsp Water

I love to vary my bath bombs to fit my mood. Start with the basic recipe and try the different ingredients below.

Uplifting

Orange and rosemary. Use 5 drops of orange and 2 drops of rosemary essential oil. Leave out the pink clay and swap the rose petals for dried orange peel and chopped rosemary leaves for an uplifting bath bomb.

Detoxing

Activated charcoal and eucalyptus. Swap the pink clay for ¼ activated charcoal and add in 5 drops of eucalyptus essential oil.

Calming

Lavender and eucalyptus. Leave out the pink clay, swap the rose petals for dried lavender heads and add in 5 drops of lavender and 2 drops of eucalyptus essential oil.

I like to make these in small batches so I can make scents that suit my mood.

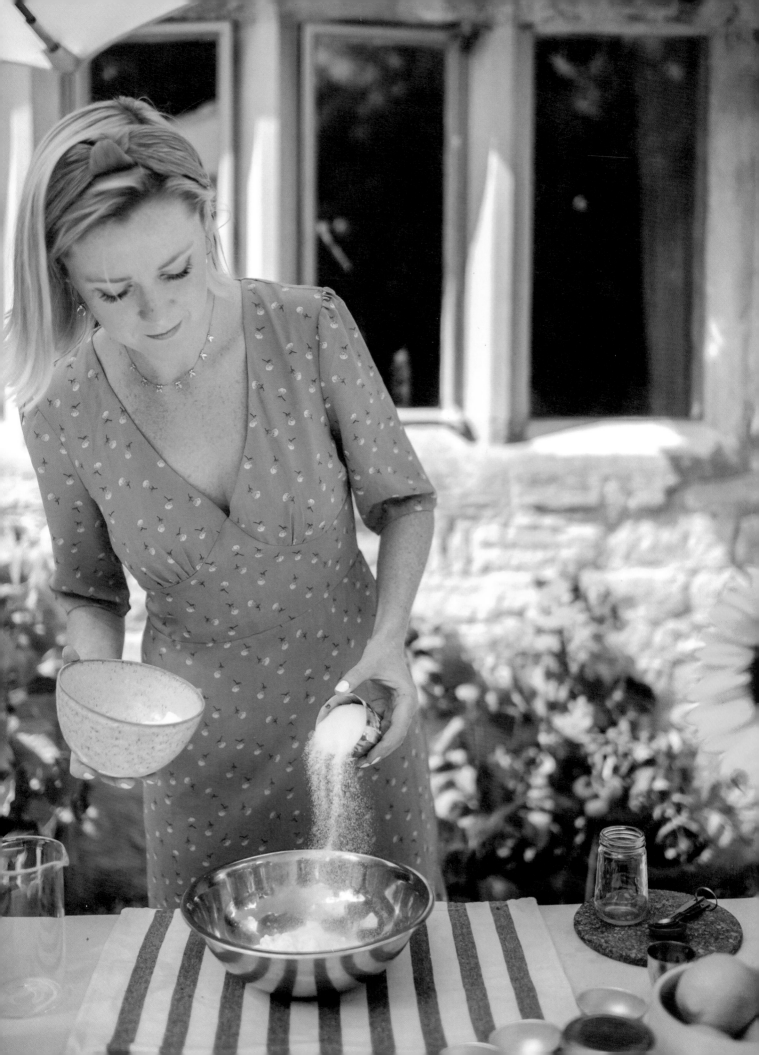

pink rose geranium bath bomb

A rose geranium is a type of geranium plant with leaves that smell strongly like roses. This species of geranium is native to certain parts of Africa. Rose geranium is used to calm anxiety and lift the spirits. It is both soothing and energising, and works beautifully to create positive energy.

What you'll need

- 1 cup Bicarbonate of soda
- ⅓ cup Citric acid
- 1 tbsp Pink French clay (optional to add colour)
- 1 ½ tbsp Dried rose petals
- ½ tsp Cocoa butter
- 7 drops Rose geranium essential oil
- ½ tsp Water

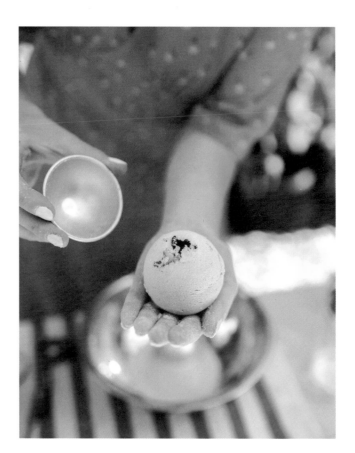

Emilie's tip

- This recipe makes ten mini bombs or 3 large ones. You can scale up this recipe or scale down to make more or fewer bath bombs; just keep the ratios the same.

Turn the page for how to make pink rose geranium bath bombs.

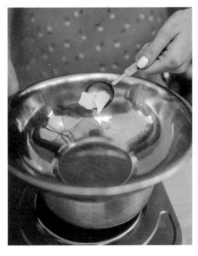

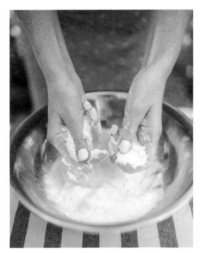

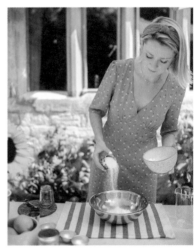

1. Measure out the cocoa butter and place it into a heat proof bowl over a pan of water to melt. Once it's melted, take it off the heat and leave to one side to cool slightly.

2. In another bowl, measure out the bicarbonate of soda and get rid of any lumps with your hands. A trick to find the lumps is to give the bowl a shake and any lumps will rise to the top!

3. Next add in the citric acid. This is what will make your bath bombs fizz when it reacts with the bicarbonate! Give it a thorough mix with the bicarb and check for lumps again too.

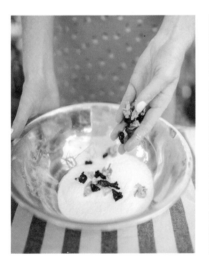

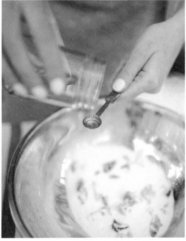

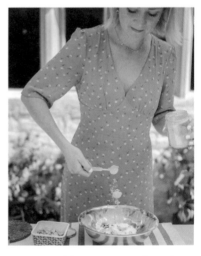

4. Add in a few rose petals for decoration, just a handful will do. I love to use my own dried petals from the garden but any dried petals will work.

5. Next you want to add in your melted cocoa butter and your essential oils. You will need to move quickly to disperse the oils in the mixture and stop any lumps forming. I find using my hands works best for this.

6. Next add in your French pink clay and mix well until evenly distributed. The clay adds colour to your bombs but will also help to make your skin feel beautifully soft & draw out impurities.

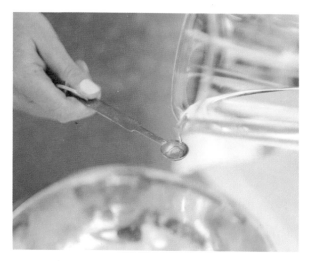

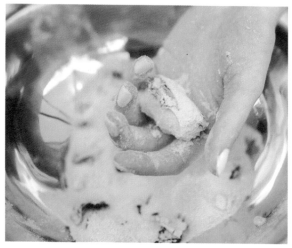

7. You now want to add in your water, little by little, mixing quickly each time with your hands to distribute it throughout the mixture. If you add too much the mixture will start to fizz & clump up, so go slow.

8. Keep adding water a few drops at a time, mixing it through with your hands and squeezing until it starts to come together and hold its shape without crumbling.

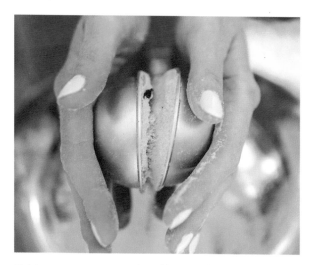

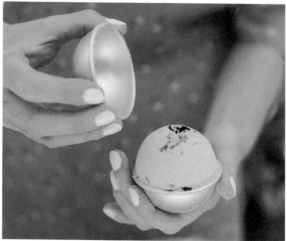

9. Now your mix is ready! I like to add a few petals to the bottom of my mould for decoration. Pack the mixture into the moulds by lightly pushing down with your fingers. Press both halves together and leave for 5 minutes before popping out of the mould to set. Don't press too hard as the liquid in the mixture will bind them together, press just hard enough to get rid of any big air pockets in the moulds.

10. After 5 minutes or so, pop your bombs out of the moulds and leave somewhere warm and dry to set overnight before enjoying!
I love to give these as gifts, just wrap up in a piece of scrap fabric & tie with a piece of ribbon.

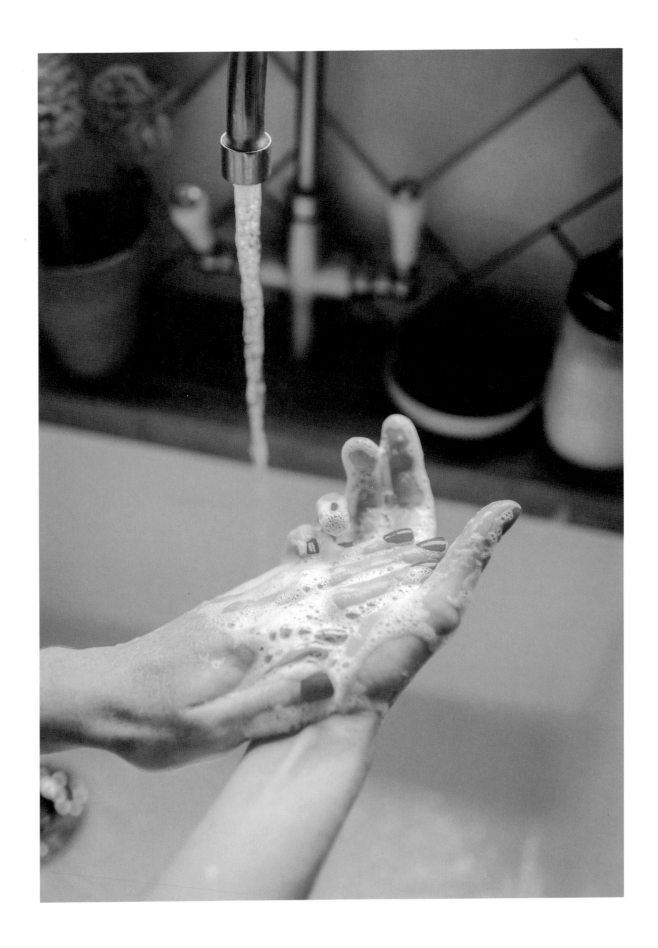

orange & bergamot foaming hand wash

A good hand wash is so important for keeping your hands supple and soft. This recipe uses a gentle plant based soap, nourishing jojoba oil and natural essential oils to add a subtle scent.

What you'll need

- 3 tbsp Castile soap
- 1 cup Distilled water
- 1 tsp Jojoba oil
- 15 drops Orange essential oil
- 10 drops Bergamot essential oil

HOW TO MAKE

1. Measure out the castile soap, jojoba oil and essential oils into a foaming soap dispenser.

2. Swirl the ingredients together until they become milky, meaning they are all combined.

3. Top up your mix with a cup of distilled water and swirl around again.

4. That's it! Your hands will be so soft when you use this soap – I recommend giving it a go straight away!

Emilie's tips

- This recipe works best in a foaming hand soap dispenser. If you haven't got one you can reuse, I'd thoroughly recommend investing in a good glass one. It will cost about the same price as a nice hand wash and you can keep refilling it with this soap recipe that costs pennies to make!

- Swap out the essential oils for your preferred scents. I like to stick to something citrus-y mixed with something a bit woodier, but floral soaps like lavender are lovely too!

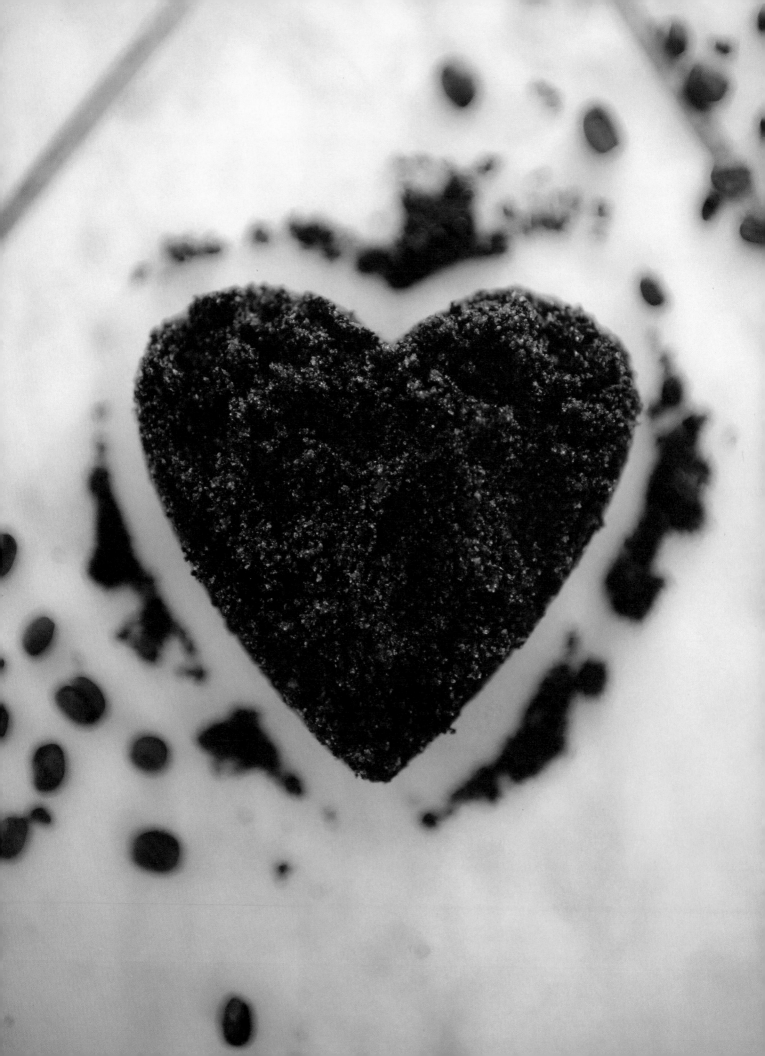

spiced coffee body scrub

This is by far the best body polish that I've ever used! It gently removes dead skin cells, whilst invigorating and brightening your skin with the sugar and coffee mix. Sugar is an exfoliator as well as a natural humectant, attracting moisture from the air to hydrate your skin. The caffeine in coffee grounds invigorate the skin, increasing blood flow which can help to reduce the appearance of cellulite. The coconut oil is also moisturising so your skin will feel so soft after using this scrub.

What you'll need

- 4 tbsp Granulated sugar
- 4 tbsp Demerara sugar
- 4 tbsp Coconut oil
- 4 tbsp Coffee grounds
- 2 tsp Cinnamon powder

HOW TO MAKE

1. Measure the coconut oil into a bowl and stir and squash any lumps with a wooden spoon to soften the oil slightly.

2. Measure the sugars, coffee and cinnamon into the bowl.

3. Mix until all ingredients are roughly combined with the oil. There will still be some lumps of coconut oil but that is okay, they will melt when using the scrub on your skin.

4. Scoop the scrub into the cooled, sterilised jar and it's ready to use!

Emilie's tips

- Apply to damp skin and scrub in circles to help remove dead skin cells, increase blood flow to the area and reduce the appearance of cellulite. When you have finished scrubbing, rinse it off with warm water and pat your skin dry. I like to use mine before I jump in the shower, it makes the shower smell like the gorgeous spiced coffee I smelt on my honeymoon in Mexico.

- You can alter this recipe to make a fantastic exfoliating face scrub. Use caster and light brown sugar instead, as these have smaller granules that are gentler on your skin. I love to use this in the morning to wake me up!

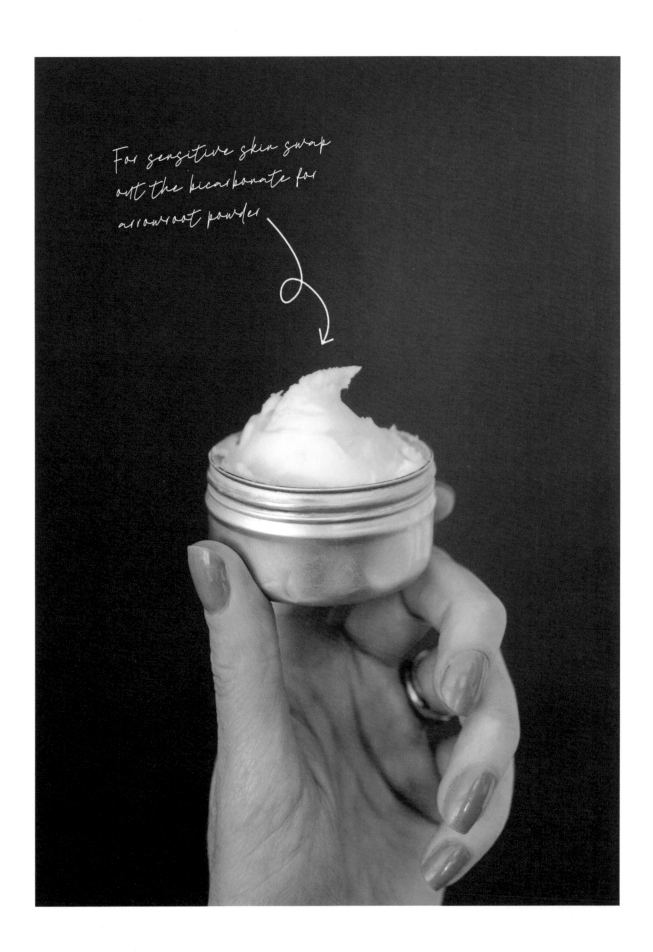

For sensitive skin swap
out the bicarbonate for
arrowroot powder

natural deodorant cream

This is my favourite DIY beauty product by a million miles. It's super cheap and easy to make, it lasts forever, its 100% natural with no nasties and best of all it really, really works.

What you'll need

- 3 tbsp. Bicarbonate of soda (deodorising)
- 3 tbsp Cornflour (absorbing)
- 2 tbsp Coconut oil (antibacterial)
- 5-10 drops Essential oils of your choice

Optional oils for a smoother texture

- Summer - 1 ½ tsp Sweet almond oil
- Winter – 3 tsp Sweet almond oil

HERE'S HOW IT WORKS

The sweat produced in your armpits isn't what smells of BO. It's actually the poo of the bacteria that eat your sweat that smells. Gross! What you need to do is create an antibacterial environment so the bacteria can't thrive in your warm, damp armpit. The coconut oil and essential oils in this recipe make a great job of this; creating an environment where bacteria can't multiply, leaving smell free armpits!

The cornflour acts to absorb any sweat that may occur and the bicarbonate of soda works as a deodoriser, in case there are some really hardy bacteria carrying on in there.

This recipe has been such a game changer for me and I'll try and get anyone who will listen to me to give it a go, so I hope you do.

HOW TO USE

Scoop out around a ½ pea sized amount of the deodorant cream and simply rub it into your armpit in the morning. If you use commercial antiperspirant at the moment you need to allow for 2-3 days for your armpits to 'detox'.

HOW TO STORE

Store in a cool dark place and try to not let the mixture melt or the ingredients will start to separate. If it does melt, don't worry, it will just need to be remixed and reset in the fridge before using again.

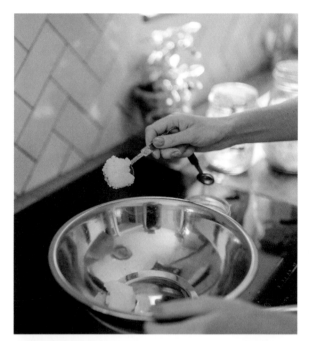

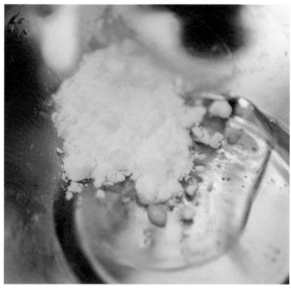

1. Measure out the coconut oil and heat in a non-plastic bowl over a pan or water until melted.

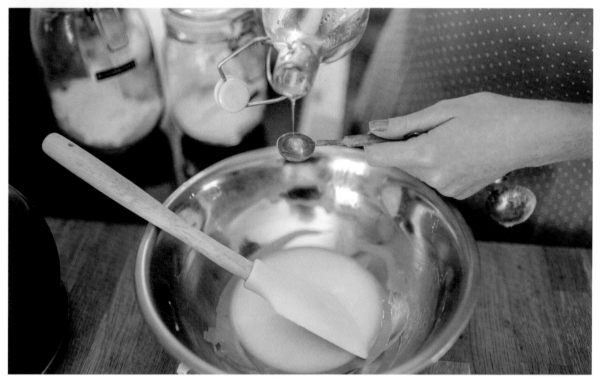

2. Take off the heat, add the bicarbonate of soda, cornflour and sweet almond oil and mix together until smooth. **3.** When combined, add your essential oils and mix again.

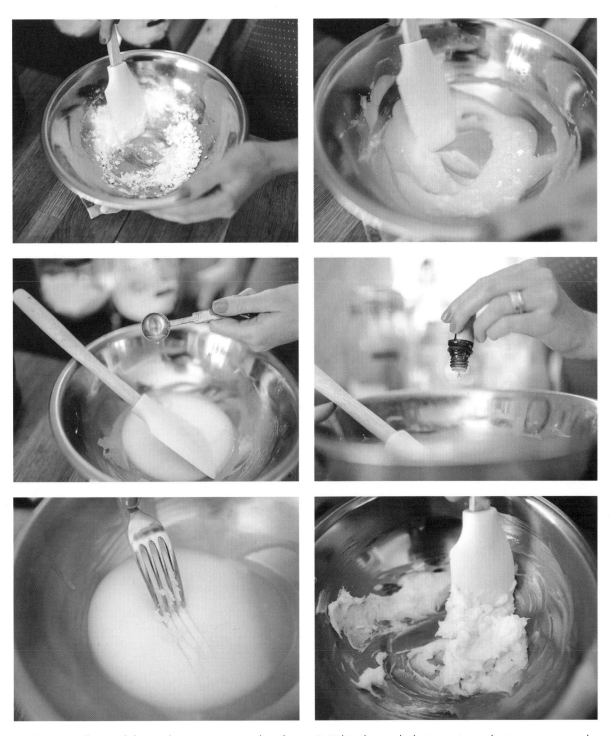

4. Once it's all smooth leave the mixture to cool and set in the fridge for 10 minutes or so.

5. Whip the cooled mixture into a buttery texture and pop into your container, ready to use!

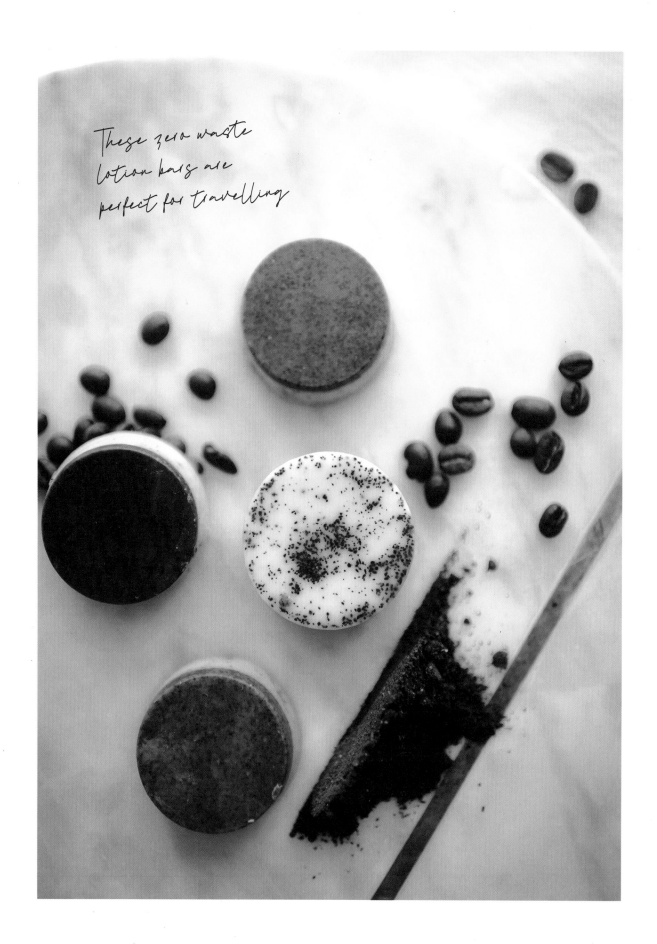

These zero waste
lotion bars are
perfect for travelling

zero waste lotion bars

Lotion bars are the ultimate zero waste travel toiletry addition, second only to the glorious shampoo bar. These little bars are quick to make, travel well in a tin or jar and are always ready to give your skin a moisturising boost, even in the shower!

What you'll need

Spiced Coffee

- ¼ cup Beeswax
- ¼ cup Shea butter
- ¼ cup Coconut oil
- 2 tbsp Coffee grounds, used
- 4 drops Cinnamon essential oil

Pink Rose & Chamomile

- ¼ cup Beeswax
- ¼ cup Shea butter
- ¼ cup Coconut oil
- ½ tsp Beetroot powder
- 4 drops Rose essential oil
- 4 drops Chamomile essential oil

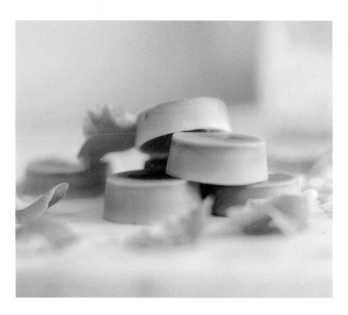

HOW TO MAKE

1. Using a bowl over a pan of boiling water, melt the beeswax and then add in the shea butter and coconut oil.

2. Take off the heat and leave to cool for 5 minutes, stirring every minute or so to stop any lumps forming.

3. Add in the beetroot powder or coffee grounds and the essential oils and mix to combine.

4. Pour the mixture into silicon moulds and leave to set overnight.

Emilie's tips

- These bars are perfect for your plastic-free travel routine! Just make sure they aren't left anywhere too warm as they could melt.
- If you don't own a silicon mould tray, muffin cases will work just as well.

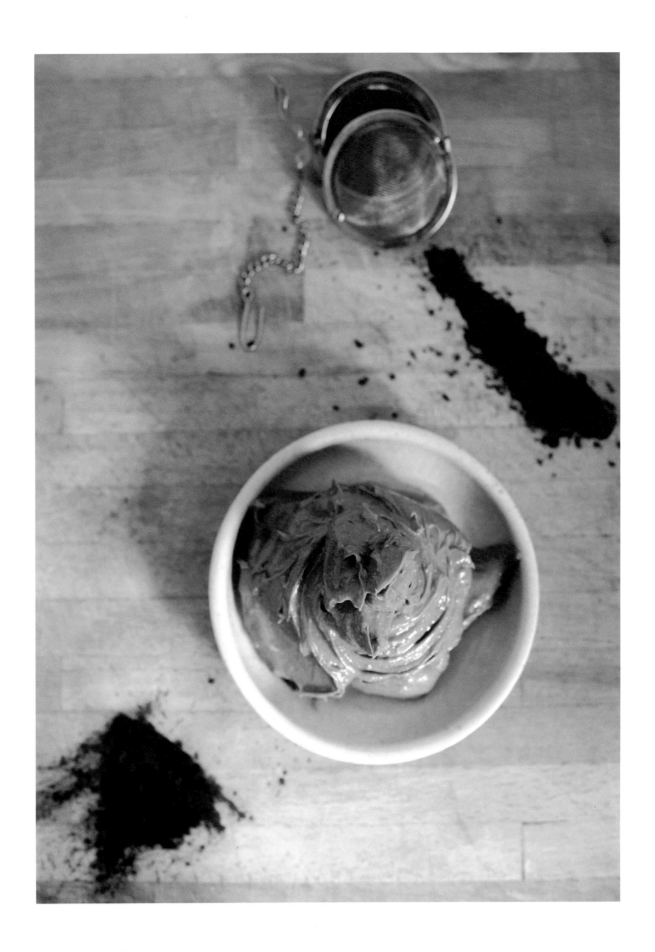

gradual tanning tea cream

I'm sure you're dubious. Tanning with tea, really? Oh, yes! This is a great natural, gradual tanner and, thanks to the cocoa powder, has a lovely subtle tint when first applied. This recipe only uses natural tanning ingredients including the tannin from brewed tea and cocoa powder, giving it a chocolatey scent.
I promise, you won't turn into an oompa loompa.

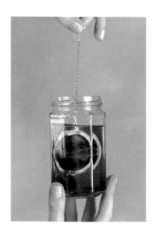

What you'll need

- 2 English Breakfast tea bags brewed in 2 tbsp of boiling water

- 1 tbsp Shea butter

- 2 tbsp Coconut oil

- 2 tbsp Beeswax

- 3 tbsp Sweet almond oil

- Cocoa powder to tint to desired colour

HOW TO MAKE

1. Brew the tea for 20 minutes or so and leave to cool completely.

2. Using a pan over a bowl of water, melt the beeswax and coconut oil before adding in and melting the shea butter

3. As soon as it is all melted, take off the heat and add in the sweet almond oil, mixing thoroughly to combine.

4. Sieve in the cocoa powder and tea, mixing thoroughly.

5. Keep adding cocoa powder until you reach your desired depth of colour.

6. Leave to cool in the fridge for 20 minutes or so until the mixture begins to harden.

7. Whip the mixture with an electric whisk until it is light, fluffy and looks like chocolate mousse.

8. Transfer the mixture into a glass jar and use within 1 month

Emilie's tips

- For a lighter tint, brew the tea for no more than 10 minutes.

- You can choose how dark you want the tint to be by the amount of cocoa powder you add.

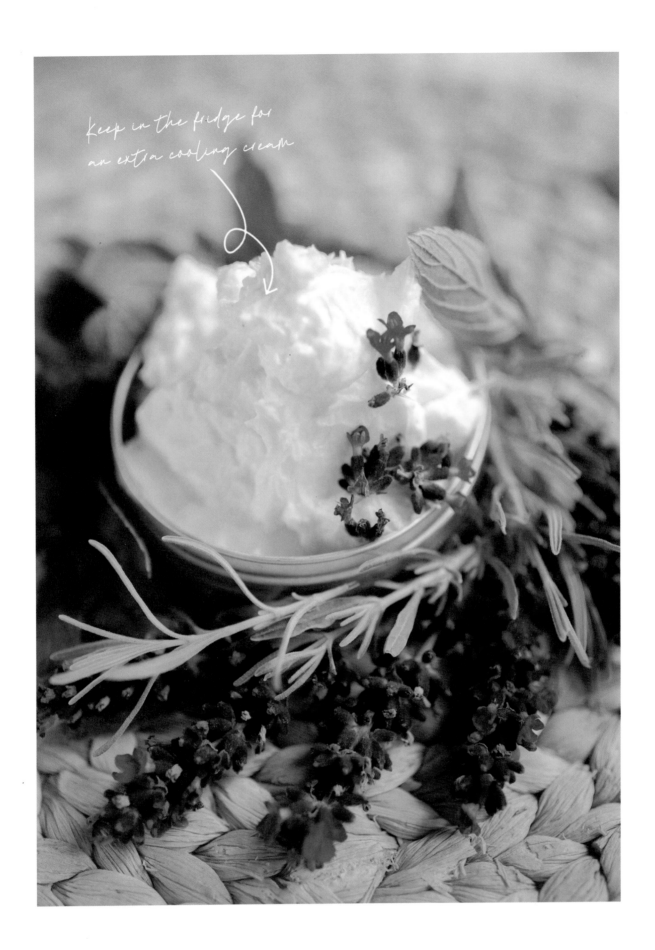

keep in the fridge for
an extra cooling cream

lavender & peppermint
after-sun cream

*As someone with fair skin, I've always relied on a cooling and moisturising
after-sun cream to help my skin recover from a day in the sunshine.
This recipe uses nourishing coconut oil, shea butter and aloe vera.
I love using it straight from the fridge.*

What you'll need

- 4 tbsp Shea butter
- 2 tbsp Coconut oil
- 1 tbsp Sweet almond oil
- 1 tbsp Aloe vera gel
- 1 tsp Cornflour
- 5 drops Lavender essential oil
- 15 drops Peppermint essential oil

HOW TO MAKE

1. In a bowl over a pan of boiling water, melt down the shea butter and coconut oil.

2. Take off the heat when melted and add in the sweet almond oil, aloe vera gel and cornflour and mix thoroughly to combine.

3. Set aside in the fridge for 10 minutes or until the mixture has begun to turn opaque.

4. Using an electric whisk, whip the mixture until the texture is light and fluffy.

5. Add the essential oils and whisk again to combine.

6. Scoop into a sterilised jar and store in the fridge.

Emilie's tip

- Lavender essential oil helps to calm and heal your skin while the peppermint essential oil helps to cool your skin down and speed up the healing process after sun exposure.

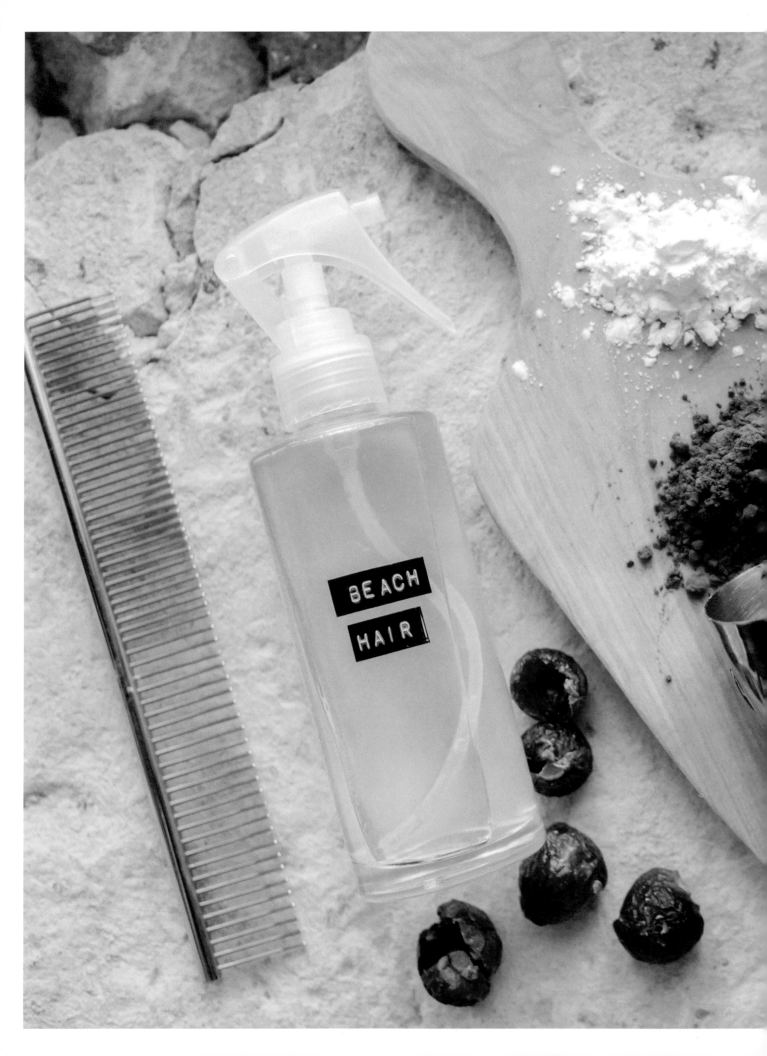

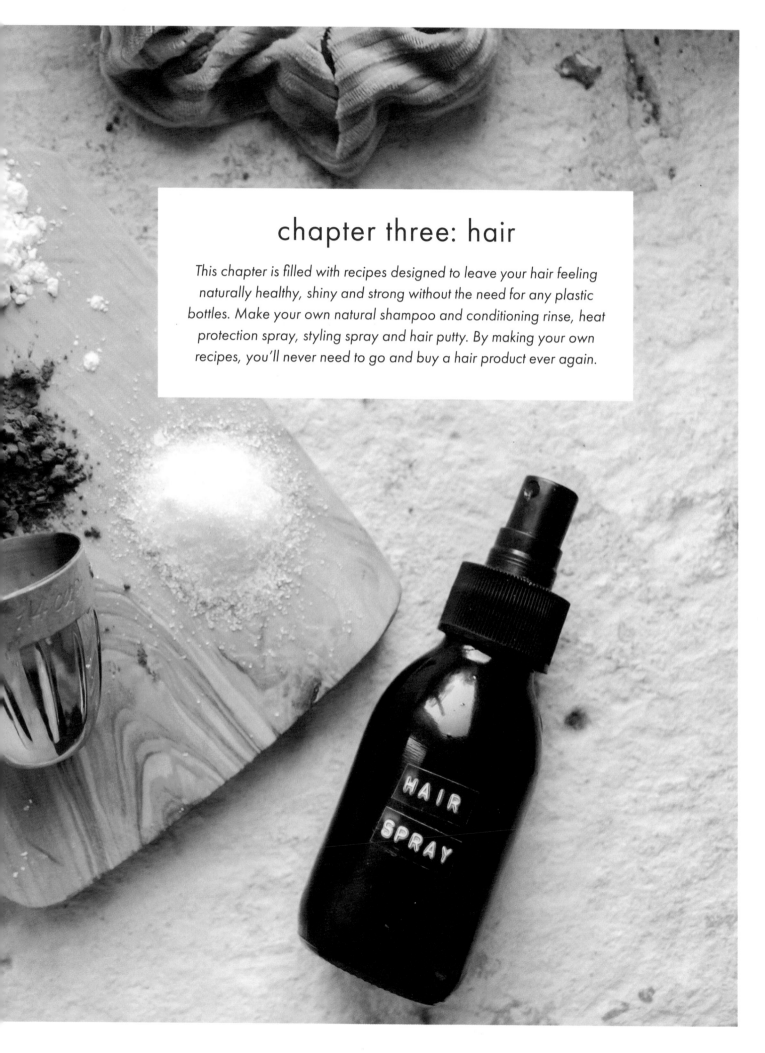

chapter three: hair

This chapter is filled with recipes designed to leave your hair feeling naturally healthy, shiny and strong without the need for any plastic bottles. Make your own natural shampoo and conditioning rinse, heat protection spray, styling spray and hair putty. By making your own recipes, you'll never need to go and buy a hair product ever again.

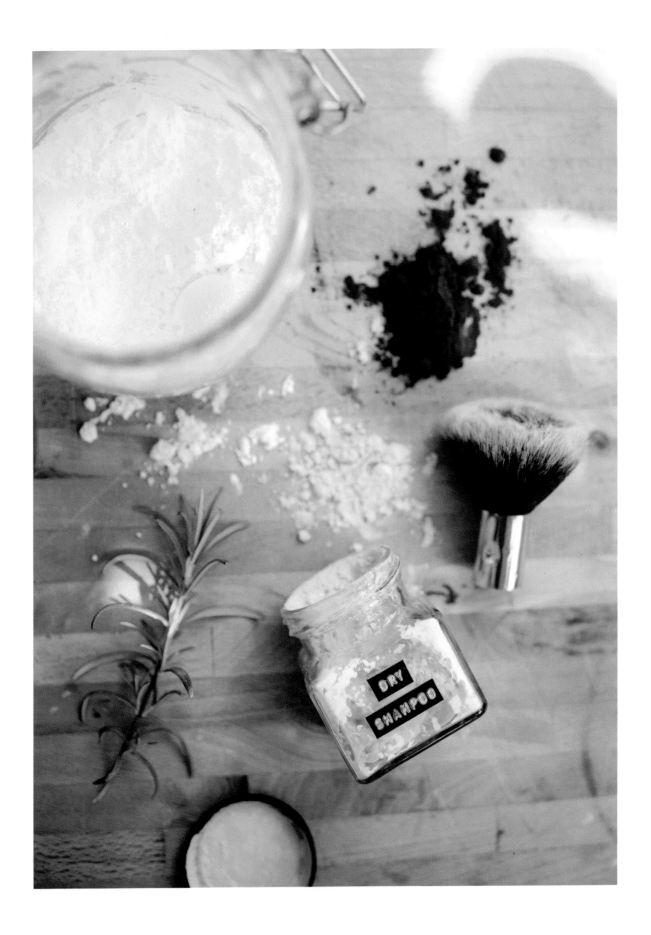

rosemary dry shampoo

This lovely scented dry shampoo lasts for ever and is so easy to make. You'll probably have the ingredients in your cupboards already! To use you just need to apply the powder directly where it's needed; it will leave your hair feeling soft, clean and not at all powdery!

What you'll need
- 2 tbsp Cornflour
- 2 tsp Cocoa powder
- 4 drops Rosemary essential oil

HOW TO MAKE

1. Measure the corn flour and cocoa powder into a small container.

2. Shake the powders together to combine them.

3. Keep adding more cocoa powder, a small amount at a time, until the colour matches your hair colour.

4. When you've created your chosen colour, add the essential oil and shake for approximately 30 seconds to evenly distribute it throughout the powder.

5. You're ready to use!

HOW TO USE

Apply by dabbing an old powder brush into the container, tapping off the excess and brushing it over your roots; working it into your scalp. Use a hair dryer to heat up the oils so they absorb quickly into the powder. This method will leave your hair feeling clean and dry and not powdery.

Emilie's tips

- This mix is perfect for my ash blonde hair. If you hair is darker, add cocoa powder until you reach the right shade.
- For red hair, swap out the cocoa powder for cinnamon.
- Old spice or sugar shakers are another great way of storing and applying this dry shampoo to your hair.

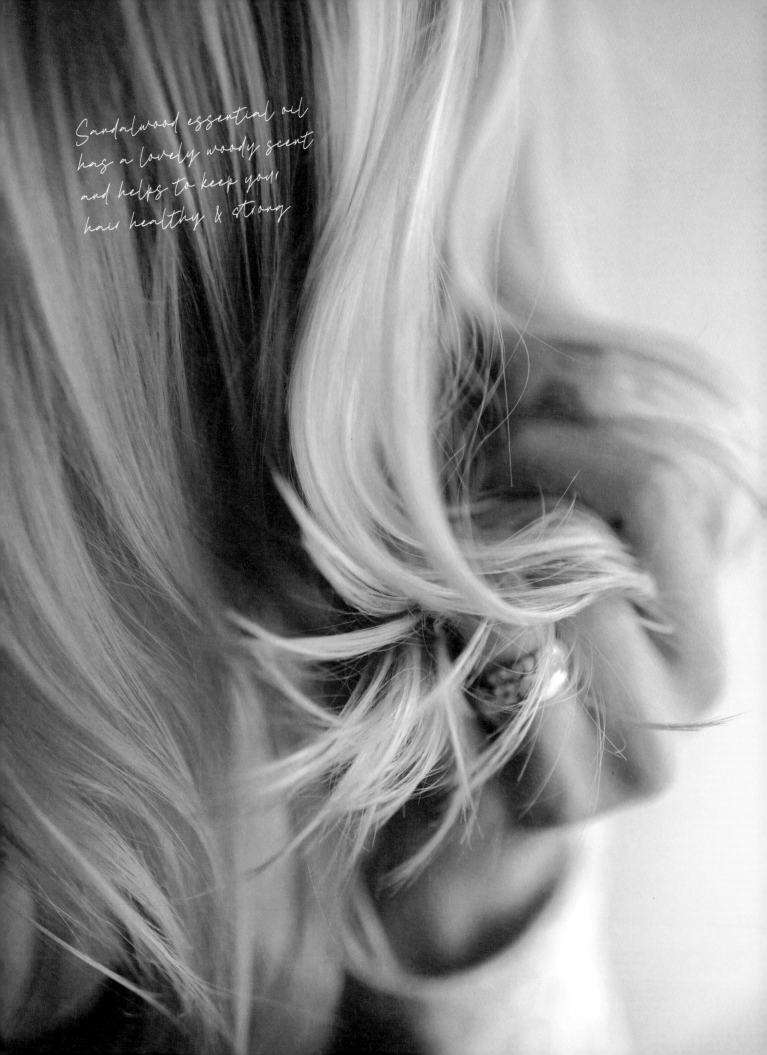

Sandalwood essential oil
has a lovely woody scent
and helps to keep your
hair healthy & strong

texturising clay

This recipe is a perfect swap if you use wax or putty in your hair styling routine and want to ditch those plastic tubs. It's a super simple, organic, natural recipe that you can adjust for the perfect level of hold for your hair. It's so quick and easy to make, I promise you'll never go back to shop-bought. All the ingredients nourish and protect your hair, whilst giving it a great hold and texture.

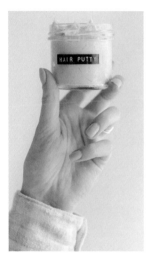

What you'll need

- 3 tbsp Shea butter
- 2 tbsp Beeswax
- 2 tbsp Sweet almond oil
- 2 tbsp Bentonite clay
- 5 drops Sandalwood essential oil

HOW TO MAKE

1. Using the double boiler method and a non-metallic pan, melt the beeswax until liquid and then add the shea butter.

2. Keep stirring, using a wooden spoon or spatula, until the shea butter has just melted, then take off the heat. Shea butter can burn and go grainy if left on the heat too long.

3. Pour in the sweet almond oil and, using a spatula, stir thoroughly to make sure no lumps are formed.

4. Add in the clay and essential oil, beating it in carefully and scraping down the sides to prevent sticking.

5. Keep beating until the mixture can hold peaks when you lift out the spatula.

6. Once the mixture is thick enough, you're ready to transfer it into your chosen container.

7. Let it sit over night to completely set. Then you're ready to start styling away!

Emilie's tips

- You can increase the level of hold of the clay by increasing the amount of wax and clay and reducing the shea butter and sweet almond oil quantities.
- Bentonite clay has been used for centuries in hair care. It is valued for its high mineral content which removes toxins and adds shine.
- Do not use any metallic equipment when using bentonite clay as it turns it toxic and dangerous to put on your skin.

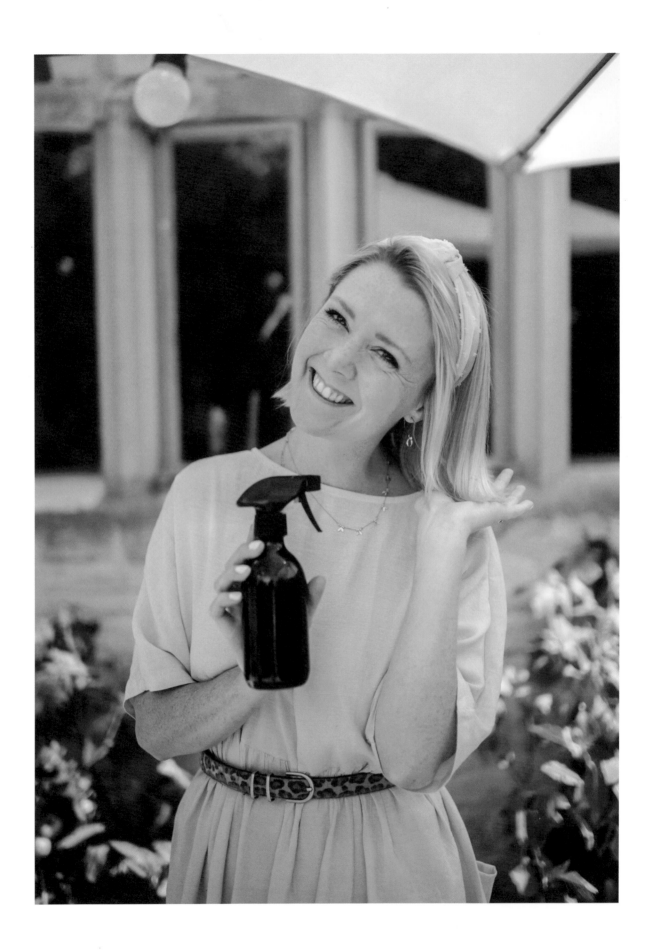

natural peppermint shampoo

Commercial shampoos clean your hair by chemically stripping it of all your natural oils. Some companies even add in plasticisers (yep, that's just our old foe plastic with a fancy name) to make your hair feel silky after using.

What you'll need

- 2½ cups Water
- 10 Soap nuts
- 2 tsp Aloe vera gel
- ¼ cup Apple cider vinegar
- 15 drops Peppermint essential oil
- 10 drops Rosemary essential oil

Emilie's tips

- You can use the discarded soap nuts as a natural slug repellent by whizzing them up in a food processor with some water to create a thick foam to put around your plants.

- The shampoo will last about a week. You can Freeze the extra liquid to use when you need a refill.

My shampoo is nothing like ordinary commercial shampoos. It doesn't lather, it's applied with a spray bottle and contains only natural ingredients. But trust me, this recipe will leave your hair feeling nourished and silky soft when it's dry. Soap nuts contain sapoin which naturally cleanses your hair and is perfect for anyone with sensitive skin. The aloe vera helps to keep your hair moisturised and balances your hair's pH to help promote healthy hair growth. Apple cider vinegar removes product build up and closes hair follicles, which leaves your hair feeling light, shiny and super soft. Turn the page for how to make your shampoo.

HOW TO USE

1. Brush your hair until tangle free before washing.

2. Wet your hair.

3. Roughly divide your hair into three sections and liberally spray your hair from root to tip with the liquid.

4. Massage it into your roots. It will feel very different to normal shampoos, but I promise it's doing great things for your hair.

5. Leave it to sit on your hair while you finish bathing or showering.

6. Rinse your hair.

7. Towel dry and brush your hair. If you find it quite tangled, spritz a small amount of leave-in conditioner or my DIY tangle spray on your hands and run through your hair.

8. Leave to dry and enjoy having naturally silky locks.

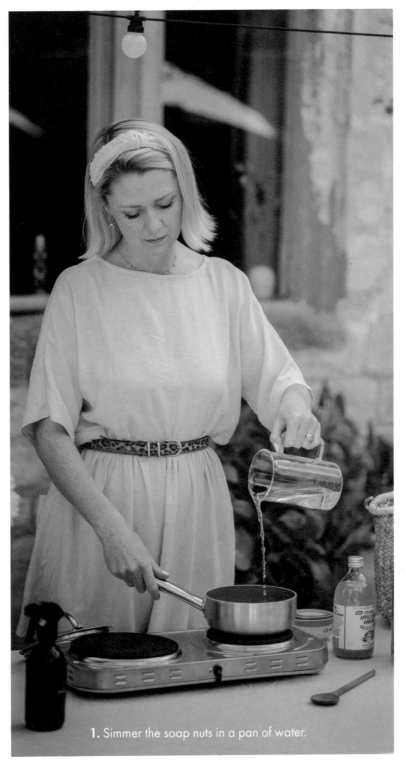

1. Simmer the soap nuts in a pan of water.

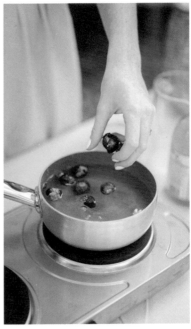

2. After 20 minutes, turn off the heat and leave the mixture to cool.

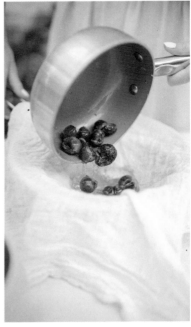

3. Drain the soup nut liquid through a muslin cloth into a large bowl.

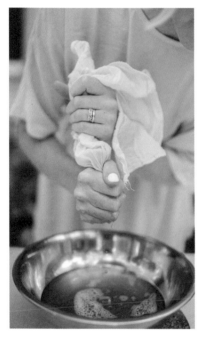

4. Squeeze the cloth until every last bit of liquid is removed.

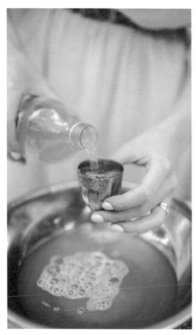

5. Add the apple cider vinegar and mix together thoroughly.

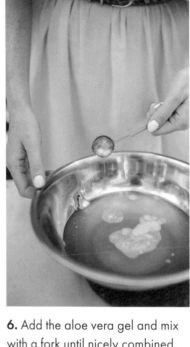

6. Add the aloe vera gel and mix with a fork until nicely combined.

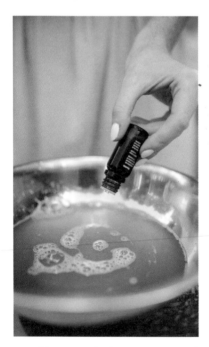

7. Add essential oils; rosemary and peppermint smell beautiful.

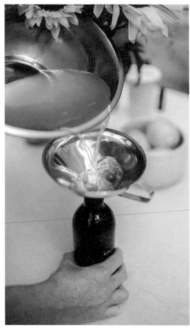

8. Decant into a clean spray bottle and give it all a good shake.

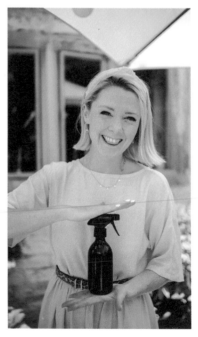

9. Your shampoo is ready to use. Freeze any extra in ice cube trays.

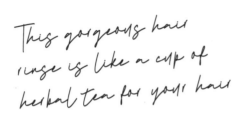

This gorgeous hair rinse is like a cup of herbal tea for your hair

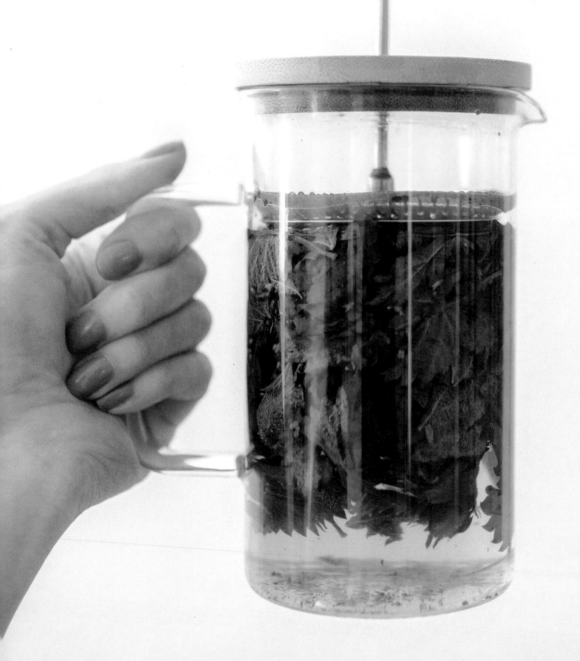

conditioning herbal hair rinse

This herbal hair rinse smooths and cleans your hair, leaving it feeling silky soft and looking shinier than ever. It helps to remove the build-up of styling products in your hair whilst smoothing down the hair follicles, to give you a light, shiny and tangle-free finish.

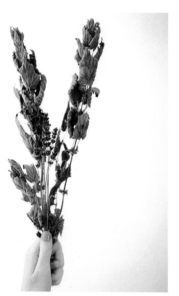 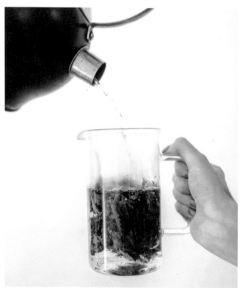

What you'll need

- 3 cups Boiled water
- 3 tbsp Apple cider vinegar
- 4 stems Nettles
- 5 Lavender heads

Emilie's tip

- To have these ingredients all year round, dry your herbs and keep them in an airtight jar or swap them for essential oils (2 drops of lavender will be enough)

HOW TO MAKE

1. Pop your kettle on to boil.

2. Strip the dried nettle leaves and lavender heads and put them, along with the apple cider vinegar, into a cafetière.

3. Pour 3 cups of boiled water into the jug and leave to brew for 20-30 minuets

4. Strain out the herbs and put them into your compost bin.

5. Store the rinse in the fridge until you're ready to use

HOW TO USE

After shampooing, pour about ½ cup over your hair and leave to sit for about 2 minutes before rinsing out with warm water.

If you don't like the vinegar smell (which won't last) you can swap it out for apple juice instead.

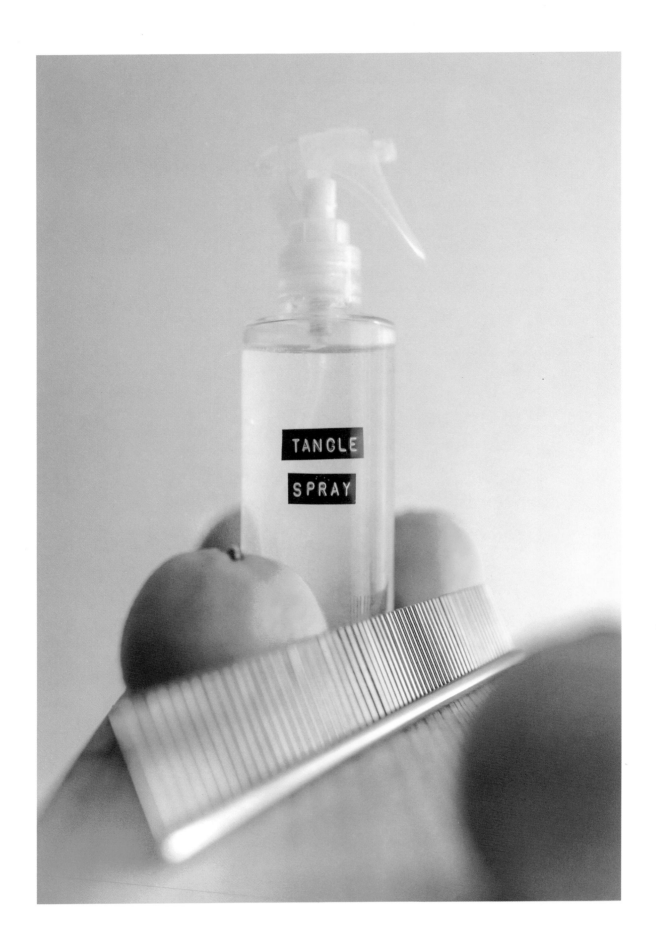

orange blossom tangle spray

For me, there nothing much more beautiful than the smell of orange blossom water, so I couldn't wait to use it in this tangled hair DIY product. Orange blossom water is usually used in baking, but has fantastic qualities for your skin and hair. It's super moisturising and gives your hair a real lustre and shine as it keeps it beautifully moisturised through the day.

What you'll need

- 1 cup Orange blossom water
- 3 tsp Aloe vera gel
- 1 tsp Glycerine

I have really fine hair that tangles very quickly, so this tangle spray is a daily product for me.

The aloe vera and glycerine used in this recipe help to add a beautiful shine to your hair, and help make it more manageable.

HOW TO MAKE

1. Measure out and pour all of your ingredients into a jug.

2. Whisk to combine.

3. Pour into a spray bottle and you're ready to go!

Emilie's tips

- This product should last around 3 months.
- I love to use this as a quick moisturising face spritz too; the ingredients are also fantastic for your skin.
- This is great for knotty kid's hair.

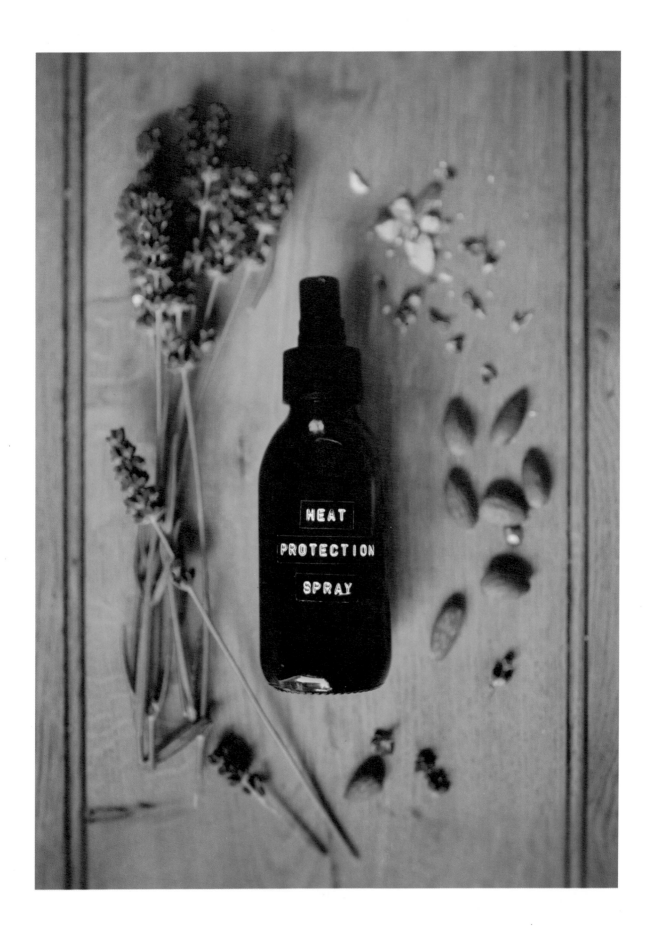

lavender heat protection spray

This spray not only protects your hair, but the essential oils and aloe vera help to make it strong and shiny. Aloe vera is particularly good for adding bounce and shine to your hair whilst providing a protective seal to keep the elements at bay throughout your day.

What you'll need

- 1 ½ cups Distilled water
- 1 tsp Sweet almond oil
- ½ tsp Aloe vera gel
- 5 drops Geranium essential oil
- 5 drops Lavender essential oil

Being someone who has fine, coloured hair I've struggled in the past with heat damage from too much straightening and blow drying. This heat spray adds a protective layer to your hair, meaning it gets hot rather than your actual hair. The oils in this recipe are incredibly nourishing and will add a beautiful shine to your locks and help prevent split ends.

HOW TO MAKE

1. Measure out the oil, aloe vera and essential oils and pour directly into your bottle.

2. Top up with distilled water.

3. Shake well before use.

4. Apply to wet hair ends before drying and styling.

Emilie's tips

- If you have **oily hair**, and want to add volume to your shampoo – add 1 tsp of salt into the mixture.
If you have **dry hair** – add in 1 tsp of glycerine to create a protective layer and help keep your hair moisturised.
For **frizzy, curly hair** – add in 1 tsp sweet almond oil to help nourish your locks.

- Reusing an old spray bottle is always best, but if you haven't got one lying around, you can use either an atomizer bottle and spray it directly onto your hair, or a pump bottle; just rub the liquid between your hands before massaging it into the ends of your hair.

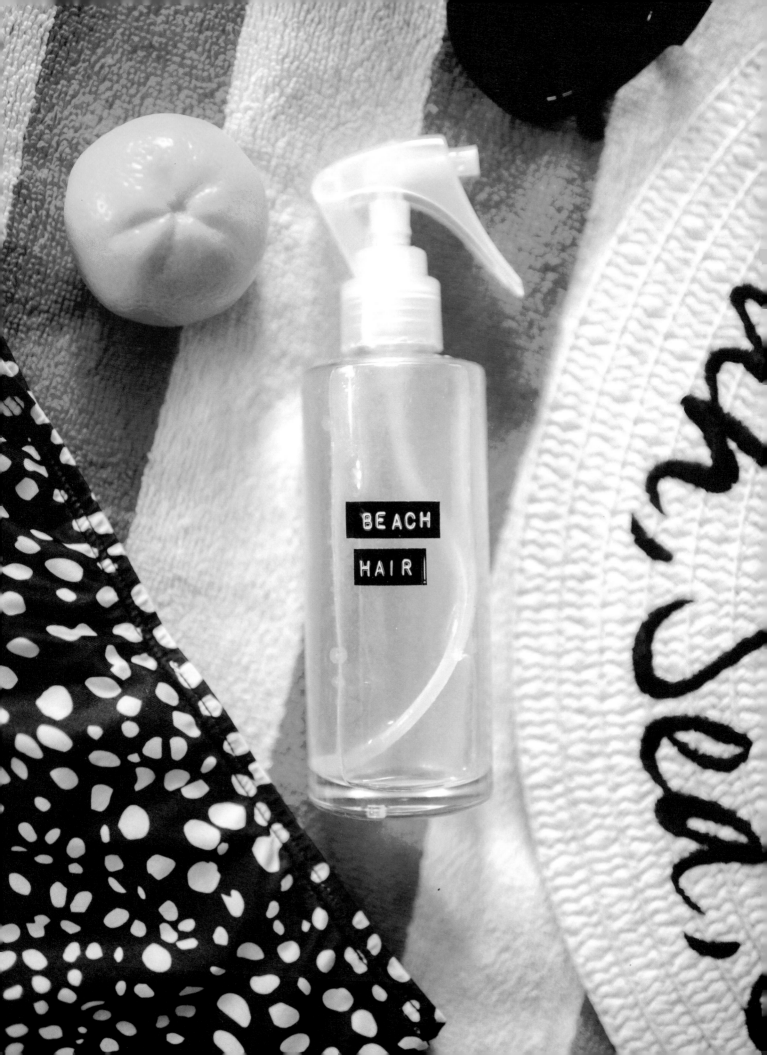

holiday beach hair spray

This sea salt spray transports me to family summer holidays in the South of France. The smell of fresh lavender and the salty sea air is just so evocative. This spray leaves your hair full of texture, volume and, best of all, smelling of holidays.

What you'll need

- 1 cup Distilled water
- 1 tsp Aloe vera gel
- 2 tbsp Sea salt
- ¼ tsp Sweet almond oil
- 7 drops Lavender essential oil

If you want that gorgeous beach waves look, this spray will create that must-have messy texture whilst protecting your hair from the sun. A touch of light lavender scent makes your hair smell beautiful and gives you a natural style that lasts.

HOW TO MAKE

1. Boil the water and leave to cool completely.

2. Measure out the sea salt, aloe vera gel, sweet almond oil and the lavender essential oil into a bottle.

3. Top up with the distilled water.

4. Shake thoroughly until the salt has dissolved.

5. You're done! Just remember to shake before each use to combine the ingredients.

Emilie's tips

- If you're using a clear bottle, add in a few sprigs of dried lavender for a lovely botanical look. It will also continue to infuse to create a stronger lavender scent and a lilac tint!

- For an extra beachy look, add in 2 tsp of lemon juice which will begin to naturally highlight your hair!

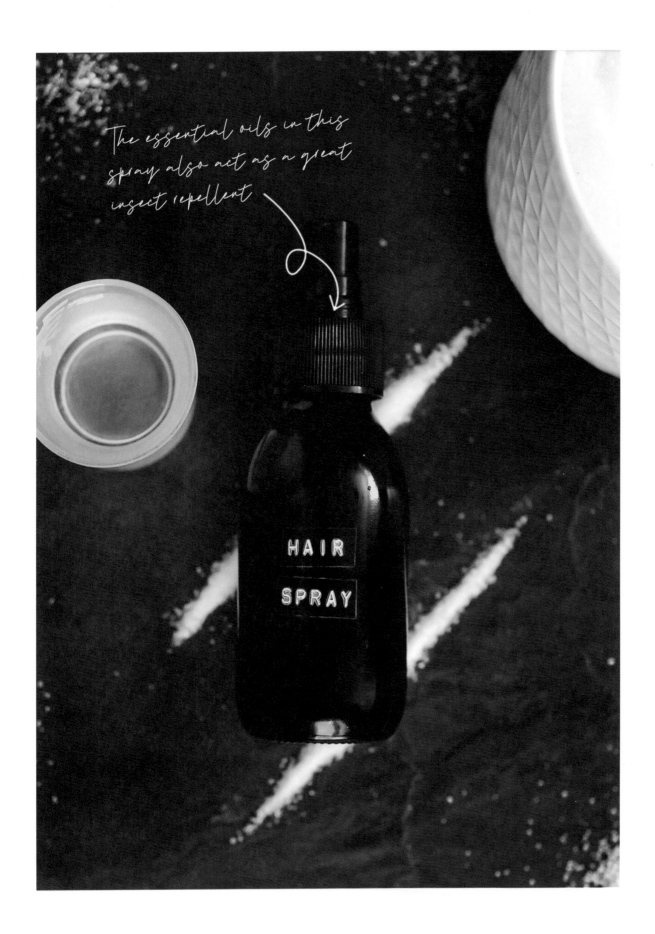

The essential oils in this spray also act as a great insect repellent

HAIR

SPRAY

rosemary sugar hair spray

I love this natural flexi-hold hairspray. The sugar attracts moisture from the air to keep your hair hydrated and silky whilst also holding it in shape. It's great for flyaways and holding in curls.

What you'll need

- 1 tbsp Vodka
- 1 cup Distilled water
- 1 tbsp Granulated white sugar
- 4 drops Rosemary essential oil

Commercial hairsprays use plasticisers which are, as you've probably guessed, our old foe with a different hat on – plastic. When you wash hairspray off your hair, those micro plastics are washed away into our oceans. So, ditch the plastic and swap commercial hair sprays for this gorgeous all-natural spray!

HOW TO MAKE

1. Pour the water and sugar into a jar and pop it in a pan of boiling water. Stir until all of the sugar has dissolved.

2. Take the jar out of the pan and stir in the vodka. Leave to cool for 2 minutes or so.

3. Pour into a atomiser spray bottle and add in the essential oil drops.

4. Shake to combine and you're ready to use!

HOW TO USE

You can use this hairspray on wet or dry hair.

Wet hair – spray all over and style as normal. You will have a silky, flyaway free finish.

Dry hair – to lock in a hairstyle or curls, spray lightly and pat over your hair for a flexi-hold finish.

Emilie's tip

- Don't worry! You won't attract any unwanted buzzy friends with your sugar spray. The Rosemary essential oil in this recipe acts as a bug repellent to keep those bees where they need to be.

hair masks

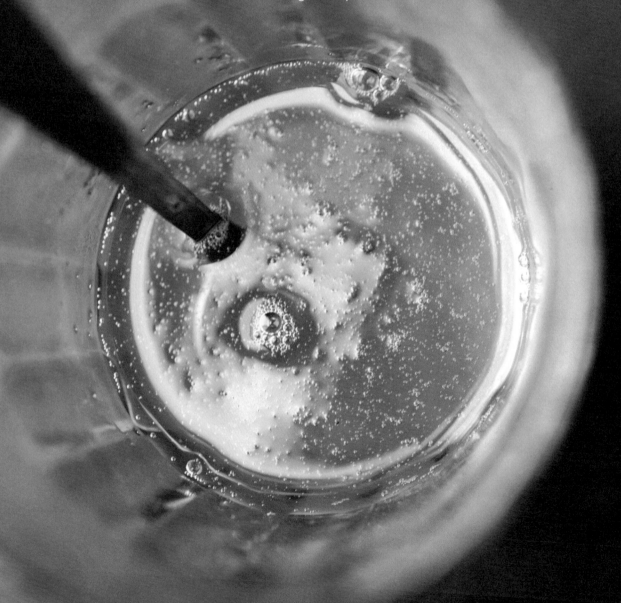

It doesn't get much more relaxing than spending some dedicated time nourishing your locks with a homemade hair mask. It's a lovely excuse to spend half an hour kicking back, reading your book and just relaxing.

Everyone's hair is different and needs different nourishment at different times of the year. With that in mind, I've created three hair masks. Feel free to mix them up with quantities to suit your hair at different times.

I hope you also feel great about never having to buy those pesky, artificial, plastic hair mask pouches ever again.
Adiós single-use plastic!

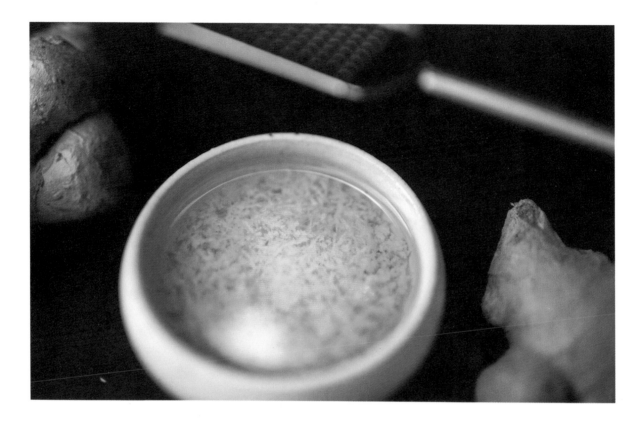

invigorating hot ginger & olive oil mask

What you'll need

- ½ cup Olive oil
- 3 tbsp Ginger - fresh grated

Emilie's tips

- I recommend using this if your hair and scalp is dry and prone to dandruff.

- Use this mask regularly, once every fortnight, for thicker, shiny hair.

This hot oil hair wrap contains fresh ginger that invigorates your hair follicles, increasing blood flow, encouraging hair growth and keeping your scalp moisturised. When applied warm to your hair, the olive oil can penetrate into your opened hair follicles, giving your hair a really deep moisturising treatment.

HOW TO MAKE

1. Heat the oil and grated ginger in a bowl over a pan of boiling water for around 10 minutes.

2. Strain the ginger out if you want a smooth mixture.

3. Leave the infused oil until you are able to handle it.

4. Smother all over your hair from root to tip and wrap your hair in a silk scarf - or a tea towel will work just as well.

5. Leave on your hair for 30 minutes before washing thoroughly with shampoo, paying attention to the roots. You may need to shampoo your hair twice to get all of the oil out.

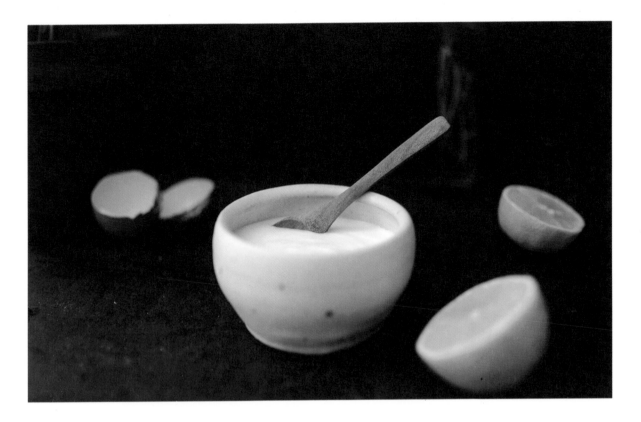

lemon & yoghurt protein mask

What you'll need

- Juice ½ Lemon

- 1 tbsp Olive oil

- 1 Egg

- 1 tbsp Full fat yoghurt

Emilie's tips

- This mask is great for dry and coloured hair that needs repairing.

- Only use this mask a maximum of once a month as too much protein can build up in your hair, making it more brittle and prone to breakage.

This protein mask works to strengthen your hair and repair the damage caused by over colouring and styling. The protein in the eggs and yoghurt work together to fortify and strengthen your hair follicles, helping to prevent future breakage.
Just pop your head over the sink and slather this mask all over your hair from root to tip. Leave it on for half an hour before washing out. I guarantee your hair will thank you for it!

HOW TO MAKE

1. Pop all of the ingredients into a bowl and mix together with a fork until fully combined. Use immediately or keep covered in the fridge for up to 24 hours.

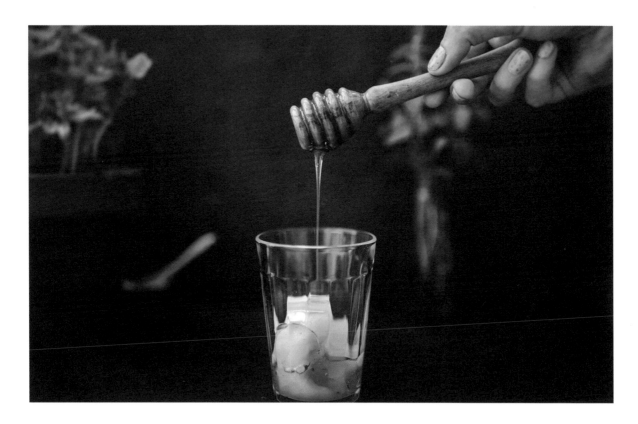

warm honey & coconut repair mask

What you'll need

■ 5 tbsp Coconut oil

■ 3 tbsp Runny honey

Emilie's tips

■ This is a great repair mask for frizzy or curly hair and hair that needs more moisture.

■ You can use this hair mask once a week.

This super nourishing and moisture locking hair mask works wonders on frizzy, flyaway hair. The honey is a humectant, attracting moisture from the air to keep your locks flyaway-free. It's great at repairing damaged hair, so focus on the ends of your hair if you have dry or split ends.

Applying this mask warm allows the hair follicles to open up, absorbing even more of that honey and coconut goodness.

HOW TO MAKE

1. Mix the coconut oil and honey together until combined.

2. Warm the mixture slightly by popping it in the microwave for 15 seconds and stirring well.

3. Apply the warm, sticky mixture to your hair, focusing on the ends.

4. Twist and clip your hair together before leaving it for 20 minutes or so to do its magic.

5. Wash out with your normal shampoo routine.

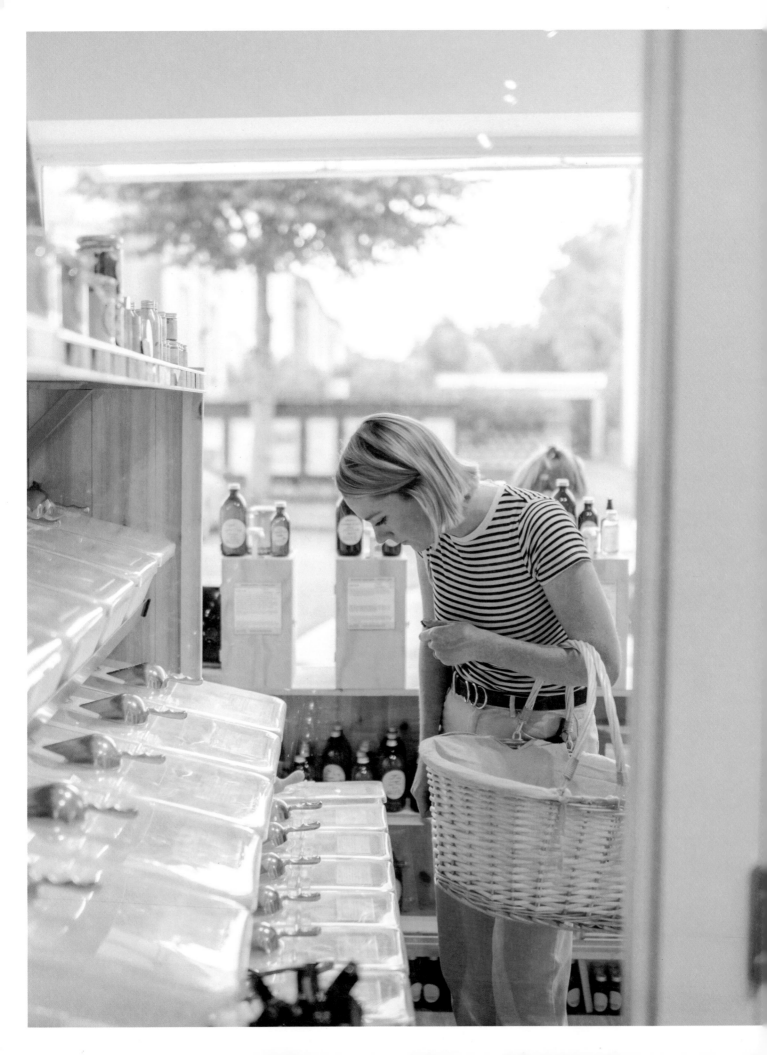

supplier directory

ONLINE SUPPLIERS
G Baldwin & Co
This shop stocks pretty much everything you'll need. From staple ingredients to more specialist ones including; essential oils, carrier oils and every kind of container you could need.

They are London's oldest herbalist and are a carbon neutral company. They do not stock any products that are tested on animals; they even refuse to stock companies who don't but whose parent companies do. All of their organic products are Soil Association approved. They are my go to for all things DIY.
www.baldwins.co.uk

Naissance
Great for ingredients & essential oils. All cruelty free and lots of Soil Association approved organic products too.
www.naissance.com

Mood Essential Oils
A great variety of essential oils online.
moodessentialoils.co.uk

Young Living Essential Oils
Beautiful high quality food grade essential oils online.
www.youngliving.com

Holland & Barrett
A great online and high street retailer for carrier and essential oils. Over 95% of the products they stock are sourced from within the UK to reduce their environmental impact.
www.hollandandbarrett.com

The Soapery
This online store has a huge variety of ingredients including butters, oils and waxes. They stock lots of organic and raw products and offer plastic-free packaging. www.thesoapery.co.uk

Neal's Yard
One of the original environmentally aware companies, Neal's Yard has beautiful essential oils and a great community of lovely consultants who are there to help you get started. Search for your local consultant or buy direct. They also offer a closed loop container return scheme in store where they recycle returns back into new containers.
www.nealsyardremedies.com

The Soap Kitchen
This online ingredient shop has the basic ingredients and the option to pay extra for plastic free or reusable packaging. They are also Soil Association approved organic suppliers.
www.thesoapkitchen.co.uk

HIGH STREET STOCKISTS
Scoop Wholefoods, Bristol & Bath
This zero waste shop is my go to in my local city of Bristol. Scoops stock everything you could need completely packaging-free and at a really reasonable price.
98A Whiteladies Road, Bristol, UK, BS8 2QY
Unit 3, The Grain Store, Rosebery Road, Bath, UK, BA2 3GS
www.scoopwholefoods.com

Loose, Stroud
This small but perfectly formed zero waste shop in Stroud has a variety of DIY beauty ingredients and all sorts of other goodies.
4 Lansdown, Stroud, UK, GL5 1BB
www.looseplasticfree.co.uk

The Green Scoop, Carmarthen
A great community focused zero waste shop stocking all sorts of beauty DIY essentials. The owner, Jess, is full of essential oil knowledge.
9 Hall Street, Carmarthern, UK, SA31 1PH
www.thegreenscoop.co.uk

BYO, Nunhead, South East London
This zero waste store in south-east London stocks all sorts of DIY ingredients, all packaging free.
147 Evelina Road, Nunhead, UK, SE15 3HB
www.bringyourownuk.com

About the author

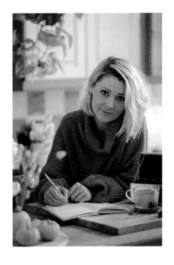

Emilie Woodger-Smith is on a mission to encourage and inspire people to live a more sustainable lifestyle. Growing up on the South Wales coast, Emilie has always been surrounded by nature. This love of nature led her to study Environmental Science at university in Bath. The more she learnt about our planet and the damage we are inflicting on it, the more she wanted to do her bit to help save it.

Emilie loves gardening, cooking and DIY and found they led to her learning to make homemade beauty products. Seeing the reduction in her waste from making her own products and the improvements in her skin, she knew she wanted to share her natural recipes as widely as she could on her blog and Instagram account.

"It can seem pretty intimidating to live sustainably, as if it's all or nothing. I aim to show you it only takes a few small changes to have a really big impact. A sustainable lifestyle really can be simple."

Blog - www.simplysustainable.living.co.uk
Instagram - @simply_sustainable_living

Acknowledgements The first and biggest thank you has to go to my fantastic husband and amazing photographer, Joab. This book wouldn't be here if it wasn't for Joab bringing me all those cups of tea to keep me going and patiently retaking a shot that wasn't exactly as I imagined. You're the best and still I love you all the stars. Thanks too to my parents for their unfaltering support for me and my dreams of making the world a more sustainable place. Starting out as a kid making fairy potions using flowers in the garden, who'd have thought I'd write a book about them! To my girlfriends who were a lifeline when I was working on this book, cheering me on without fail and testing out dodgy fledgling recipes to help me perfect them - thank you for being my guinea pigs. To my inspiring aunty Lorna, who was the person that started me off on my DIY journey, sparking my passion by sharing her homemade products and recipes with me. I wouldn't have ventured into this world of DIYs if it wasn't for you! Lastly to Honey, my crazy, lovely little pooch. All those stinky kisses, snuggles and chin rests really did help. I'm sure you knew I needed them. Love you, good girl.